What Works With Fathers?

Trefor Lloyd
Working With Men

Published by Working With Men
320 Commercial Way, London SE15 1QN

© Working With Men 2001

Layout, Design and Printing by RAP, Clock Street, Hollinwood, Oldham, Lancs OL9 7LY

ISBN 1 900468 06 9

What Works With Fathers?

'There is no correct way to engage fathers.'

(Richard Fletcher).

Acknowledgments

This piece of work was funded by the Family Policy Unit of the Home Office and we not only thank them for funding, but also for repeatedly showing their commitment to fathers and this area of work.

We would, of course, like to thank all of those projects who gave up their time to help us get the best descriptions of their work on paper and the fathers who added their comments and experience of these pieces of work. Also, we would like to thank Richard Fletcher (Men and Boys' Project, Newcastle University, Australia) and David Bartlett for reading and commenting on the first draft of this report.

This publication is dedicated to Alan Richardson, who worked hard to understand and develop appropriate services for fathers in the last few years of his life.

Contents

Introduction   9

What Works? – literature   10

Introduction to practice   21

Blackburn and Darwin Fathers' Project

(primary health care setting, working with fathers suffering from depression, and using a social care model)

Families Need Fathers, National

(support and advice network for those fathers going through divorce and separation, using a self-help and 'buddy' system)

Mancroft Advice Project – Young Fathers' Group, Norwich

(young people's advice and counselling setting, offering a support group for young fathers, using an educational and therapeutic model)

Man Enough, Oxford

(Adult Education setting; courses for fathers wanting to improve their parenting skills, using a discussion-based model)

Men United, Nottingham

(Family Centre-based, providing a support group for mostly single fathers, but also using a community development model)

NEWPIN Fathers' Project, South East London

(Parenting project-based, offering longer term therapeutic support to a broad range of fathers)

Pen Green Family Centre, Corby, Northamptonshire

(a broad range of 'gender-based' initiatives targeting fathers, mothers, children and staff within a Family Centre setting)

Rugby Parents' Centre, Rugby, Warwickshire

(Parents' Centre-based courses targeting local fathers wanting to improve their fathering skills using a discussion and educational approach)

West Wiltshire Family Centre, Trowbridge, Wiltshire

(Family Centre-based, using a discussion-based model, targeting fathers whose children have contact with Social Services agencies, including child protection)

YMCA 'Dads and Lads', Plymouth, Devon

(sports-based setting, offering football for both fathers and their children as a route into fathering issues)

Emerging themes 75

Summary of findings 88

Appendix 1 89

Appendix 2 91

Introduction

Work with fathers is a relatively new, but rapidly expanding area of work. With a range of Government initiatives, particularly through the Family Policy Unit (Home Office), The Teenage Pregnancy Unit and Sure Start all encouraging the development of work with fathers, projects are expected to mushroom.

However, just because there is funding doesn't mean that work with fathers will develop easily and smoothly. Fathers are becoming more involved in their children's lives; more mothers are in the workplace; family responsibilities are changing in an increasing number of families, but this has not necessarily led to large numbers of fathers rushing out to get involved in fathers' groups, early years provision or their children's schools.

Generations of mothers looking after their children, while fathers bring in the family income, have left a set of attitudes and beliefs (for families and childcare workers), which will take time to change; however, fathers' initiatives will have to develop in parallel.

This report has been specifically written to assist those who want to develop initiatives, but have little or no experience of working with fathers.

Over the last 25 years, there have been scattered pieces of practice, usually developed by those who felt passionately about the role of fathers, with these initiatives often disappearing as workers left or volunteers became involved in other activities. They have rarely been recorded, let alone evaluated (although this is not unusual for new areas of work that are also often poorly funded or unfunded).[1]

This report starts from the assumption that those wanting to develop new pieces of work can learn from existing practice. *What Works with Fathers?* has three parts:

a) a brief review of literature that says something about developing practice;

b) descriptions of 10 well-developed pieces of practice with fathers;

c) an analysis of these pieces of practice, with the common themes pulled out and offered as important considerations for those wanting to develop work with fathers.

What Works? – literature

This is not intended as a full literature review; that has been done, and much better than we could do it.[2] What this publication is concerned about is practice, and the literature related to practice.

This section aims to highlight practice themes and signpost the reader to significant research and publications. Existing literature is often written by researchers or practitioners suggesting areas or approaches for consideration. We have pulled out themes of significance, either aspects common in the literature, or those that are just insightful and help shed light on how work with fathers might be developed.

a) Approach fathers positively

Alan Richardson suggests we need to challenge the negative stereotype of the father which seems so pervasive ... the standard image of the father as feckless and irresponsible.[3] He goes on to suggest that these attitudes affect both fathers and the agencies trying to work with them.

Richard Fletcher makes a similar point: If we want [fathers] to get involved, we will have to do things differently. This means going after men, but it also means valuing men, fathers, for what they might contribute. It may seem an obvious point, but if we want fathers involved then it would be a good idea to let fathers know that they are appreciated and valued.[4]

However, his emphasis is in a slightly different place to Richardson's: Not that schools have said bad things about fathers, but because the normal school routine does not rely on fathers to interact with the students, fathers are easily left out of the picture.[4]

Fathers' visibility is a recurrent theme; a positive approach means, in part, making fathers visible. In contrast, accepting their absence as normal is increasingly seen as part of a negative approach to fathers.

Fletcher also suggests: Appreciating fathers is not the same as saying 'Dads are Great!' or organising a card for Father's Day once a year. Appreciating fathers must start from a positive view of the fathers in the community, but it entails actively encouraging fathers to be involved with their own children's schooling and with other students at the school.[4]

While Richardson advocates a positive approach, he also suggests this is different from rose-tinted glasses:

... as men, we need to openly acknowledge the damage that some men do inflict on *children, to challenge the abuse, to work with the abuser. But as a way of counterbalancing these front page presentations of abuse and reminding professionals that not all men are abusers, so also we need to publicly celebrate the love that many fathers bring to the nurturing of their children.*[3]

Of course, when fathers were problematic, the reasons to work with them were because they were a problem. Their fecklessness and irresponsibility meant that they were absent (physically, and emotionally), dangerous (physically for the mother and children) and we needed them to change for the safety of others. When they didn't come forward (to be worked with), it was then assumed that they didn't care about their children (or were resistant to change) and this in itself reinforced the negative view of fathers.

The new positive approach has focused on the benefits for children, the fathers themselves and mothers, indeed all of the family and society as a whole.

While this more positive approach towards fathers has increasingly influenced developing practice, it has also raised questions about what would motivate fathers to engage with their children and agencies.

b) Fathers are of benefit to their children and children to their fathers

A recent study by Charlie Lewis[5] highlighted the benefits that fathers bring to their children's social, economic and psychological development.

From a review of current literature, he concludes that men have a particular set of gendered roles (economic, play, link to the outside world), but that there is much more that is common between mothers and fathers (bond similarly, have the same capacity to love their children) and that they have the same potential for caring and supporting their children's development. Lewis also suggests that many fathers take the role of 'reserve' carers, taking up the role when mothers are unwilling or unable.

Michael Lamb suggests that *whether the outcome variable is cognitive development, sex-role development, or psycho-social development, children seem better off when their relationship with their father is close and warm. In general, the same is true in the case of mothers, and children who have close relationships with both parents benefit greatly.*[6]

James Levine places this positivism in a broader context: *Whether men are connected to their children, as well as how they interact with them, is influenced by a variety of factors, including the expectations men have of themselves and the expectations and support they have (or don't have) from family and community members.*[7]

The assumed superficiality of fathers' relationships with their children has also been questioned. Kyle Pruett suggests: *That men and children can affect each other as profoundly as any relationship that they will ever have in their life is a truth many young fathers do not understand and many older fathers hold as a canon.*[8]

Levine has suggested that the commonly held beliefs about men need to be questioned at the most fundamental level: *Contrary to stereotypical belief, men's sense of personal happiness and satisfaction is more strongly linked to their family roles than to their work roles.*[7]

This positive approach towards fathers has brought into question, what many now believe to be fixed stereotypes of fathers' behaviours and attitudes towards children and family life.

c) Fathers are already motivated to be better fathers

Graeme Russell has suggested that if we understand the relationship men have with their children, this will better inform us about the motivation men may have to be involved in services: *Fathers want to do a 'better' job of being*

a parent, especially with their sons; if they are separated or divorced; or are experiencing difficulties in their relationships with their partners. There are more too who are in-tune psychologically with the changing expectations of fathers. They want to be more involved and have a better relationship with their children than their fathers had with them, but don't necessarily want to conform with expectations about the 'new fathers'.[9]

This questioning has emerged largely because gender roles are changing, and no more so than within the economy. More women are in the workplace, while more men are in the home. The traditional breadwinning father, earning enough for himself and his family, is in decline, while families where both parents are working are increasing, as are families where mothers are the primary breadwinners.

This changing landscape means that the number of statements we can make about gender roles have also dramatically decreased, and studies have indicated that while families are changing, attitudes are lagging a little behind.

The British Survey of Attitudes indicates that younger mothers and fathers living a life where they are both bringing money into the family, are also beginning to share domestic and childcare responsibilities; however, these changes are still relatively slow.[10]

d) Some professionals' attitudes need to change

Mary Ryan has argued that professionals too often operate on traditional gender role assumptions and fail to recognise (or accept) that changes have or are occurring. She goes on to suggest that *we are still suffering the left-overs of the role of men to be economic providers, and for women to be carers*; and goes on to say:

The attitudes of professionals are crucial. In practice, it appears they almost invariably target services at mothers; many are clearly ambivalent about engaging with fathers, and evidence suggests that many actively avoid them....from the father's point of view, he readily senses how he is being 'defined out' of the childcare equation. This can, in itself, reinforce his marginalisation.[11]

e) Many fathers' attitudes are changing already

While some professionals fail to recognise these changes, many fathers do: *Virtually all of the fathers acknowledged their role was changing and that they were not sure exactly what that role was changing to; many of them said they felt less skilled (in childcare) than their partners.*[11]

f) If the problem is to be solved, we have to know what the problem is

When fathers were 'feckless and irresponsible', then it was obvious that the reason they didn't use services was that they didn't care, and they didn't think about their children. With a positive approach towards fathers, the problem is harder to identify. Some have (as we have seen above), moved the focus of the problem onto professionals, because they are thought to exclude, marginalise, and inhibit the participation of fathers.

Professionals are thought to place barriers in the way of fathers. There is certainly enough evidence to suggest that this happens; however, there is little point in moving from 'feckless and irresponsible' (blame the father), to a barrier-producing professional (blame the professional).

The reality appears to be more complex than this. Yes, Fletcher is right, we have to appreciate and value fathers' contribution, and Richardson is right, we have to acknowledge 'the damage that some men do inflict on children', and we also have to recognise that gender roles are changing (reflecting the workplace) and that men are generally reluctant users of services, especially support services.

g) Let's not forget that fathers are men first

Role theorists have suggested that *masculine roles involve a set of expectations for task-orientated behaviours that emphasise logic and rationality and de-emphasise emotional experience. From early childhood, boys come to value masculine traits and behaviours and devalue feminine ones.*[13]

Too often fathers have been looked at in isolation of their maleness. Their beliefs and attitudes about fatherhood will inevitably be, at least in part, determined by their beliefs and attitudes towards being a man. So, for example, if men are 'taught' to be strong, not to complain, not to be a wimp, then this will make it harder for men to go to their GP, because they will perceive this as weak, whinging and wimpy!

These attitudes and behaviours are reflected in the way that men use health services, where they appear to leave intervention much later than women. Fewer men go to visit their GP, and those men that do, visit less often than women; in fact, for every visit a man made, a woman made 2.1.[14]

Many men have much more difficulty asking for help. Good[15] found that men felt they needed to be in control and self-sufficient, which often stopped them from asking for external help. Balding[16] – in a survey of over 20,000 young people – asked: 'If you wanted to share health problems, to whom would you probably turn?' He found that 12.8% of 12-year-old boys answered: 'No one' (with only 6.9% of girls answering similarly), and, by 15 years-of-age this response had risen to 13.8% (5.8% of girls).

When asked: 'When you have a problem, what do you do about it?', 18.8% of 12-year-old boys answered that they 'do nothing'. Briscoe[17] *suggests that from an early age, girls become orientated towards seeking medical care for a wide variety of complaints, whereas boys learn to disregard pain and avoid doctors; hence an association is formed between being feminine and being more concerned with health.*

Research has shown that the male gender role leads men to ignore their health needs, so we can also assume that men will have difficulties asking for help in other areas they may be struggling to deal with, such as fatherhood. We will see below, that men who have attended fathering programmes and services, often come forward when it is an emergency – some services have accepted this and offered 'casualty' for men as their point of entry into an agency.

h) We appear to have three separate and related components in working with fathers

i) professionals' attitudes towards fathers, that may be influenced by outdated notions of the father's role within the family and pre-occupation with negative beliefs about fathers;

ii) fathers' reluctance (as men) to look for help and assistance in the rapidly changing role of being a father;

iii) a relatively under-developed picture of fathers' actual role, of the benefits to children of fathers and what motivations will need to be harnessed.

i) Men do not attend services, but why?

Adrienne Burgess and Sandy Ruxton have suggested: *The traditional explanation has been that fathers are unwilling to attend (services) and there is indeed evidence that fathers tend to endorse the role of mothers as chidcare experts. Fathers, for instance, attend child health clinics when requested by their partners or when there is a 'serious' developmental issue to consider.*[18]

So they can do it, but as substitutes for the real carer, or when they are needed in the role. Kathy Weingarten questions this when she says the problem is about fathers' competence: *We desperately need to make the case for creating conditions that allow fathers to be* as competent as mothers. *It is adequacy, not just absence, we desperately need to address.*[19]

j) How do we get fathers to attend services?

Graeme Russell has suggested a number of guiding principles that summarise elements of this positive approach to fathers:

- fatherhood is expressed in a diversity of ways;

- both women and men have potential to be competent parents;

- the majority of fathers have strong feelings towards their children;

- under most circumstances children actively seek to know, identify with and have acceptance from their fathers, and benefit from fathers reciprocating in this relationship;

- presume that fathers and mothers have shared responsibility for children;

- balance between paid work, family involvement and intimacy in relationships has potential benefits for the well-being of fathers and their families;

- fathers can experience difficulties in being assertive and finding the space to be as involved as they would like (or to have their contribution recognised and valued);

- fathers value and respond to the experience of sharing their concerns with other men;

- focus on 'what is in it for fathers?';

- some fathers have accepted the challenge to confront traditional expectations and have been highly effective in changing their own lives.[9]

k) Are fathers' groups the answer?

Russell has stressed the importance of understanding what motivates fathers to reflect on fatherhood and want to develop their skills. However, he believes that this does not necessarily mean that fathers will be queuing up for fathers' classes.

Taken from an extensive study of fathers, he found 'the majority of men are concerned about their future roles as fathers, want to spend more time with their children and would seek parenting support, but that only 15% of men would consider joining a fathers' group.[9]

Emma Longstaff also makes the point that fathers' groups have their place, but also limitations: *It is important to note that fathers' groups may not fit many working men's lifestyles. For these men, bringing fathers' groups or workshops into* *the workplace, or developing programmes that include activities with their children, may be one solution.*[20]

Longstaff also found that many fathers were reluctant and nervous about attending fathers' groups: *When asked how they had felt when first coming to a meeting, words such as 'dubious' and 'sceptical' were used, and more frequently 'uneasy', 'anxious' and 'bloody terrified'.*[20]

These comments suggest that we need to look wider than fathers' groups, and that maybe the questions we need to ask as practitioners are: 'What can we do to enhance fathers' involvement in their children's lives?' and 'What can we do to enhance fathers' work generally?'

Unfortunately, inexperienced practitioners are more likely to ask: 'How can I recruit for a fathers group?', without really thinking through whether a fathers' group is the appropriate answer to the fathers' question!

We will return to this issue but, not surprisingly, most fathers' projects have highlighted targeting and recruiting as the major barriers to their development, and Longstaff found that most fathers who attend fathers' groups described:

- isolation as lone parents;

- desperation of marital break-up and separation; or

● children's behavioural problems as their primary motivation for attending.[20]

She reinforces the need to identify primary motivation, saying that: *Levine and others have observed, certain moments in fathers' lives offer golden moments for intervention, such as the birth of a child or, more unhappily, divorce. Agencies who have contact with families at these times should be certain to make the most of these golden opportunities, and design their services accordingly.*[20]

l) What can professionals do to enhance fathers' involvement in services?

Mary Ryan in her study of fathers within social services environments makes a number of recommendations that emphasise the need for professionals to act to remove barriers for fathers. She says that *professionals should 'ask and not assume' what role the father(s) and any father figures play in the family…collecting information on the family's circumstances should be done routinely. This should include information about the fathers and/or father figures, whether they are resident in the home or not.*[11]

She is critical of the professional focus on mothers. She says: *If professionals do not attempt to find out about or engage with fathers, partly it is because fathers distance themselves. This is not a problem specific to social services but applies to other agencies working with children and families as well.*[11]

She suggests that *there should be a presumption that working with and engaging the father will benefit the child, but careful assessment in individual cases will identify the circumstances where attempts to engage the father by social work staff would be counter-productive.*[11]

Deborah Gharte et. al. explored both fathers' attitudes and experience of family centres and of staff's attitudes towards fathers. Interestingly, Gharte concluded that there were three different approaches to working with men/fathers:

1. centres that regarded men and women users as the same … often reported fewer barriers (at least as far as staff were concerned), tended to be enabling – but only for certain groups of men. They were often used by men in 'special' orientations to fatherhood, but less so by other men;

2. centres that regarded men and women users as 'different' … were often very conscious of the problems of working with men, but because they were actively engaging with these 'problems' and differences, also tended to be relatively enabling; and

3. centres that took what we called an 'agnostic' approach – that is, they didn't really seem to have a view … (these) tended to be associated with the greatest number of barriers reported by staff and parents, and often the least number of enabling factors. In short, these seemed to most feminised and the least 'father-friendly'.[21]

This suggests that awareness and consideration of gender is important for professionals to enable them to engage fathers effectively. Gharte goes on to make some very valuable distinctions between the fathering role and men, and suggests that many family centres have difficulties because fathers are indeed men!:

Yet where men were concerned, our data suggested that some centres seemed to have difficulty with allowing men in 'on their own terms'. Indeed, it sometimes seemed that men were welcome in family centres only as parents, and not as men in their own right. Few centres offered any activities of interest or appeal to men.

She goes on to recommend:

The first and most important change necessary would be to **reduce the level of female dominance within family centres**. Centres would need to encourage more positive, accepting and actively welcoming attitudes towards men in women users and staff, and in particular discourage women from giving vent to the kind of anti-male sentiments.... and

The second area for change would be a **positive commitment on the part of centres to recruit men**, backed up by action – and persistent action at that.

m) Are fathers' groups enough?

Interestingly, Gharte is one of those authors who strongly encourage a multi-dimensional approach:

We concluded therefore that though men's groups are enabling for some, they may not be a first line of service provision. Providing a men's group alone is unlikely to be a successful way to recruit large numbers of fathers. Rather, men's groups should perhaps be viewed as an 'advanced' activity for established users of centres.

n) Who attends fathers' groups and why?

There have been two attempts to analyse who attends fathers' projects, what the fathers get out of them and what approaches may work. Alan Richardson drew up tentative typologies or frameworks for fathers' work, based on his audit of fathers' projects in the North East of England. While Richardson suggests that:

It might be tentatively speculated at this point that different types of groups attract different types of fathers, with different types and levels of personal issues and concern about their fathering activities and approaches.[3]

He poses some important questions if we are to understand why and which fathers attend services.

He also explores the approaches used

by projects to engage fathers, finding that either projects are *experimental (and open in nature) or (use a) structured didactic approach (shorter, time-limited), although some pieces of work straddle various categories, and as a group develops may move from one category to another. He suggests that neither way is 'right'; different ways of engagement and working have to be devised to suit the different codes of language and communication styles of the men participating with the group.*

Burgess and Ruxton have suggested there are four (sometimes overlapping) models that have developed:

● socially based, usually meeting with their children and involving trips out;

● behaviour-based programmes, where men's abusive behaviour is usually the main focus;

● a more educationally-based format, where childcare skills and parenting dilemma's and problems (such as smacking and discipline) are a central component;

● therapeutically-based groups where discussion, personal experience, education and sometimes masculinity are strong elements.[18]

o) Different horses for different courses

Richardson, while analysing the facilitation style, also raises important questions about whether these approaches are themselves a barrier to participation.

This relationship between motivation, targeting and facilitation will be returned to later, because it is such a central issue to developing work with fathers. Richardson quotes David Bartlett (while at NEWPIN) *when he said that once the ice is broken, it is surprising how eager the fathers are to talk.*

This suggests that those fathers who get themselves into fathers' groups are either fine and open once they are in this setting, or self-selecting, being men who are open to the approach, before they arrive. This again will be a theme explored later.

In this brief review of practice related writings, we have tried to pull out those issues that tell us something about what works with fathers. Not what works in fathers' groups, but what works with fathers. Having read much of the recent literature, we almost know too much.

The various studies had lots to say about fathers, their motivation, what they think are important, etc. What we have tried to do is to focus on the core of what works, and what practitioners need to address to enable them to develop work with fathers effectively.

References

1 Caddle, D. (1991) *Parenthood Training for Young Offenders: an evaluation of courses in young offender institutions*. Home Office Research and Planning Unit, Paper 63. HMSO, London.

2 Lamb, M. (ed) (1997) *The Role of the Father in Child Development is one rare exception*. Wiley, Chichester. Graeme Russell, Charlie Lewis.

3 Richardson, A.J. (1998) *An Audit of Work with Fathers throughout the North East of England*. Children North East, Newcastle-Upon-Tyne.

4 Fletcher, R. (1997) *Getting DADS involved in schools*. Family Action Centre, The University of Newcastle.

5 Lewis, C. (2001) *Father Facts*.

6 Lamb, M. (ed) (1997) *The Role of the Father in Child Development*. Wiley, Chichester.

7 Levine, J. with Pitt, EW. (1995) *New Expectations (community strategies for responsible fatherhood)*. Families and Work Institute, New York.

8 Pruett, KD. (1987) *The Nurturing Father*. Warner Books, New York.

9 Russell, G. Barclay, L. Edgecombe, G. Donovan, J. Habib, G. & Pawson, Q. (1999) *Fitting Fathers into Families*. Commonwealth Department of Family and Community Services, Australia.

10 British Social Attitudes Survey (1992) HMSO, London

11 Ryan, M. (2000) *Working with Fathers*. Radcliffe Medical Press, Oxford.

12 DIY Dads, (1999) *Consultations with Fathers*, Working With Men.

13 Kilmartin, C. T. (1994) *The Masculine Self*. MacMillan, New York.

14 Lloyd, T. (1998) *Men's Health – a public health review*. Men's Health Forum, London.

15 Good, G. E., Dell, D. M., Mintz, L. B. (1989) *Male Role and Gender Role Conflict: relations to help seeking in men*, J. Counselling Psych. 1989; 36(3):295-300.

16 Baldings, J. (1993) *Young People in 1992*. Schools Health Education Unit. University of Exeter.

17 Briscoe, M. E. (1989) *Sex Differences in Mental Health*. 1989, 834-839.

18 Burgess, A. & Ruxton, S. (1996) *Men and their Children: proposals for public policy*. Institute for Public Policy Research, London.

19 Weingarten, K. (1994) *The Mother's Voice*. Harcourt Brace, New York

20 Longstaff, E. (2000) *Fathers Figure: fathers' groups in family policy*. Institute for Public Policy Research, London.

21 Garte, D. Shaw, C. & Hazel, N. (2000) *Fathers and Family Centres: engaging fathers in preventive services*. Policy Research Bureau, London.

Examples of practice

To arrive at the ten examples of practice, projects had to be selected. Initially, 23 projects were identified (see Appendix 1) as established fathers' projects that had been in existence for at least two years and had worked with a substantial number of fathers.

Projects were initially contacted to see whether they were interested in being involved. Fifteen replied, and these were then looked at in terms of geography, types of settings, and styles of work, to ensure that the broadest variety of projects were included.

Unfortunately, some projects either just did not reply (even though they were phoned or written to on at least six occasions), or they said that they could not be involved. (This was either because staff had moved on and the work was at a very low ebb or had completely disappeared, or that circumstances such as staff illness, being inspected or other pressures made the commitment difficult.)

Projects were then visited between October and December 2000, although three interviews were carried out over the phone because of the rail network and weather problems during this period. Background information was also used and fathers involved in the initiatives were spoken to, usually on the phone after the visits. Drafts were then prepared, returned to the agencies for comment, with the descriptions below having been agreed with all of the projects involved.

Trefor Lloyd
Working With Men

What works? – Blackburn and Darwin Fathers' Project.

During 1994 whilst working as a counsellor at a Doctor's surgery in Shadworth, Richard Edmonds became increasingly concerned at the number of men suffering from depression, and lacking in confidence in their own ability. He noticed that they were all fathers. With the support of the Shadsworth surgery, he applied to the local Health Authority for funding to set up a fathers' group.

Limited funding was received in April 1995. Richard had identified a number of fathers who were long-term sick, socially isolated and clinically depressed, who he was already counselling individually, and they were invited to the group, the aim of which was to 'help them to begin to feel that they could have a positive role.'

This would be done by providing them help to give each other mutual encouragement and assistance with parenting skills and also to 'help them to develop their relationships with their own children's.'

Richard talked to each of the fathers individually, and five of them were interested. All of these were aged 30-40 years, white, one had four children under 10 and two had children in their early teens. Most had experienced hospitalisation for their depression.

When he spoke to them, they all voiced concerns about the Summer holidays, how they would entertain their children, how they could do this cheaply, etc. Richard therefore started the group with trips to local parks (including picnics) with their children and helped them identify places and activities that they could do with their children.

This was followed up with Friday morning meetings in a local Neighbourhood Centre, dominated by what Richard describes as 'chat and a brew'. He says he was trying to 'create an atmosphere which was comfortable, informal and enabled the men to talk'. Richard saw his role as an enabler.

With isolation being so pronounced for this group of men, he thought it very important that they talked to each other and got involved. There was pool, dominoes and a TV and on the first Friday of the month; everyone sat down for a meal which they prepared themselves.

Richard says that a more formal approach would not have worked for these men. Discussions about fatherhood were also informal, and usually initiated by the fathers themselves. He believes that the fathers became more confident through their participation, less depressed and that it also impacted on their diet (and their children) through the monthly meals.

After the first year, Richard says that 18 fathers had been through the group, although numbers were usually five or six for each session. Some men left the area, while others got jobs. Different activities have been introduced: a Christmas Party was organised by the fathers for their children. The organising process increased their confidence and brought the men closer together. Trips out, picnics and an allotment all provided the fathers with opportunities to work together and increase their confidence.

In a 3 year review, Richard writes:

'Looking back over three years, I have seen a steady growth in the work. Over 50 referrals, coming mainly from GPs and also health visitors, schools and self-referrals.

It is important working at Primary care level that no stigma is attached. I am currently involved with 25 dads; the number of dads referred is constantly growing. I mostly deal with long term issues: disabilities, physical and mental illness. Clinical depression is one of the major problems coming through the surgery door, plus community depression, fear and intimidation.'

Support for the dads is two-fold:

● building up mutual support and encouragement i.e. weekly meetings;

● build-up of the informal support network.

It has been very encouraging seeing the gradual build-up of support in these areas.

Richard says that a variety of issues emerge from the men about their fathering role which include:

● a dad worried about his girlfriend who has post-natal depression following the birth of her child (who has Down's Syndrome);

● a dad who lost his job because he had extended time off to look after his family during his wife's complicated childbirth; and

● a dad who is seeking access to see his own children (his solicitor has offered free legal advice to other dads in the group).

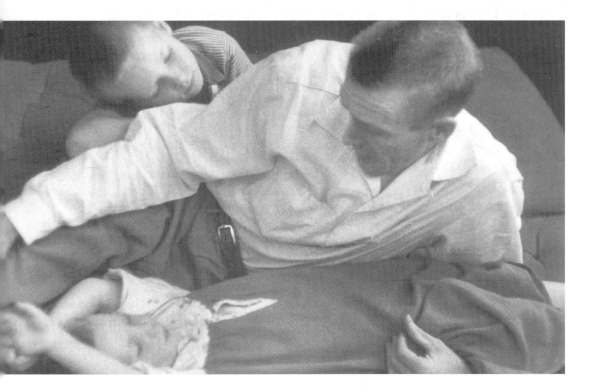

Since becoming involved in the group, some men have grown in confidence enough to get involved in community associations, go to college and improve their literacy. For many, they are getting more involved in their children's lives, especially taking them out and doing things with them.

Richard is of the view that the group has met three important needs for these men:

● they feel valued, and see their role (as fathers) as important and it has increased their confidence;

● it has provided a regular and stable environment where the men could socialise, and use it as a starting point for further community involvement, and;

● it has given focus to their individual educational needs and has provided a place to make friendships with other men similar to themselves.

Plans for the future include a Sure Start extension to the current group in a nearby area, Sudell.

This description was based on a conversation with Richard Edmonds, a number of reviews and articles written about the group. Richard was unable to give us contacts of men he was working with. Richard can be contacted on 01257-462550, or 12 Wood Lane, Parbold, Wigan, WN8 7TH.

What Works? – Families Need Fathers

Families Need Fathers was formed in 1974 and provides information and support to parents, including unmarried parents, of either sex. FNF is chiefly concerned with the problems of maintaining a child's relationship with both parents during and after family breakdown.
What FNF say they do:
we work to increase awareness of the problems of family breakdown;
we produce booklets, leaflets, a website and a regular newsletter;
we provide speakers and case studies for the press and media;
we collate and promote relevant research information;
we participate in family policy forums and seminars;
we lobby Parliament and the legal profession;
we provide support to members through our online information exchange; and
we have a network of volunteer telephone contacts and local branches.

Most people who know of FNF will be aware of their lobbying work, their outspoken positions on fathers, or the occasional controversy (World in Action accusations of supporting abductions or the view that they are a crowd of misogynists).

What fewer people will be aware of, will be that 90% of their work is support work with parents (mainly fathers). This aspect of their work is in three forms, monthly (or bi-monthly) local meetings where men can talk about their situations and get advice and support; phone help from a nation-wide volunteer network (45 are listed in 'McKenzie', the FNF two-monthly membership magazine) and a members'

chat room linked to their very impressive Website (on www.fnf.org.uk).

Annual membership is £25.00 and FNF has a current paying membership of 3,000 plus (which has been growing steadily by 10-15% for the last few years, and this is expected to continue).

The local support meetings started in 1975 with 'Walk In Talk In' at Conway Hall in Central London. Trevor Berry (one of the founders) says that 'on a good night there were 10 fathers, one chap took the chair and the rest sat around'. Trevor is of the view that the form the meetings take has changed very little, they are just bigger.

He says that all kinds of friendships

have developed, even fathers exchanging houses for the weekend when they have children in towns where the other lives. There are currently 19 meetings nation-wide every month, chaired by volunteers and open to anyone. The Central London meeting is held in a room of a Holborn pub, every Tuesday evening.

Here are my observations of one of those meetings:

There were probably more than 50 men (and three women), with at least 12 of these there for the first time. The meeting was chaired, the chair asking first timers to talk about their circumstances, and then the chair would give advice and comment. Other men would give their experience and comment on strategy.

The men's circumstances were desperate: breakdown of contacts; mothers who use drugs and prostitution; court agreements which were not working; children seriously at risk; and men who had not seen their children for some while. There was no hesitation for men to talk, in fact there was a queue!

All of the men who spoke had already had contact with the court system and solicitors. All had run out of ideas, had not got what they expected from the court system and did not know what to do next. They had become disillusioned with the courts and complained that the courts were 'unfair'.

Richard explained parental responsibility and other basics and tended to comment on 'how the law operates' and not the law itself (which, of course, was appropriate for a self-help group). He, but particularly others, gave advice about strategy: 'keep calm, don't go over the top', 'you will have to collect evidence', 'the judge won't take that into account', 'you will need to make sure that they know about ...'

There were certain statements made that brought noises of agreement and approval: 'the courts are unfair, they do not treat men well', 'you can't trust the legal system (or solicitors) to fight your corner' and that 'you have to be very smart, and strategic'.

Most of the men who asked for advice and those who gave it, were very articulate, with the tone usually being direct, but supportive. Those who gave advice, took the testimonies on face value, did not question the details and responded to the situations offered.

Because of the desperate positions men were in, the advice given could have been preparing these men for war. 'Watch your back' and 'remember, you could be killed out there!' would not have been out of place in the comments made from the floor. We heard no 'anti-women' comments or advice given, with the 'baddies' being seen as solicitors and the court system.

I think, the combination of desperate situations, and the kind of advice given, as well as the meeting being held in a pub, and self-help, all contributed to the obvious appeal of these advice sessions. There was an appropriateness of tone and gravity as well.

Most of these men had to be desperate before they would seek advice. If someone had said: 'What about mediation?', most people in the room would have laughed, and quite rightly.

While the main meeting was going on, in a nearby side room a barrister gave individual advice; a queue formed for this additional service, and a steady stream of 'customers', sometimes gone for 20-30, minutes quickly formed.

From this visit, and conversation with Jim Parton (who is the current Chair of FNF), a number of themes emerged about the men who use these services. Many of the men are desperate, have run out of ideas and find that there is very little help, by the time they contact FNF. Jim says that they are often shocked about the court system and that they expected it to be more 'even-handed'.

Men also arrive at meetings thinking 'they are the only one'. My observations were thought to be fairly typical of those that attend; there were a lot of suits (Central London office workers) and a high level of articulation. There were a small number of African Caribbean which reflects current membership.

With an organisation financially dependent on membership fees, this also means that members have to be willing and able to shell out £25.00 a year (£20 if by Direct Debit or £10 if unwaged). Jim said that the majority of men contact FNF via radio programmes, the press and agony aunts, and was of the view that 'while we get more enquiries from mentions in the Sun, we get more joining from articles in the Mail, Guardian, Independent and the Telegraph'.

Jim also said that specific stories often bring a good response. An Express headline saying that Bob Geldoff's next big campaign was dispossessed fathers brought over 500 enquiries.

Jim is of the view that benefits for the men include: a lot of knowledge about what will happen in the court system; hard nosed 'para-legal' advice; emotional support; and the reassurance that they are not the only one.

Organisations of this kind obviously have their downsides as well. A volunteer-based service working in such a difficult area often means that emotions interfere. Jim says that some of their most energetic volunteers are still in the thick of their own cases, and their advice can be seriously tainted by this. Many of the men, as Jim puts it 'go through a mysoginistic phase', where comments about one woman easily become 'all women'.

Since becoming chair three years ago, Jim has tried to deal with 'the angry, firebrand wing' of FNF, but admits this has been difficult: 'you can't sack a volunteer', and in such a loosely structured organisation, it is difficult to monitor the activities of individual members from Cumbria to Cornwall. FNF employs one full-time and two part-time workers, who service the current membership.

Training volunteers to do both phonework and chairing meetings just does not happen. Again Jim admits that FNF support work is very good in places and very poor in others, and some of the 'good' volunteers too often 'burn out'.

Interestingly, Jim says that over one-third of all enquires come from women. Often grandmothers and sisters of men, and it is not unusual for women to be seen at meetings, and some mothers have also been offered the services provided by Families Need Fathers. FNF aims to 'provide information and support to parents including unmarried parents, of either sex' and believes that 'children have a right to a continuing loving relationship with both parents' and that 'children need to be protected from the harm of losing contact with one parent.'

What the fathers said:
Recruitment

- When I was in court for the divorce, I saw a leaflet on the noticeboard for FNF, this was back in 1988. I phoned up and went to a meeting because I still had the financial settlement and custody to agree.
- I heard a radio show on GLR, they were talking about different situations and I got a lot of ideas from that. I had never been to a men's group before, but this was really important, so I had to go.
- I heard of FNF from a radio programme and they were my salvation.

About the service

- When I went to the meeting I found that I wasn't the only one, other men had similar circumstances and some were much worse off than me. I got moral support and help with arguments. I think I may have had a nervous breakdown without their help. Sometimes men at the meeting hit a negative note which can be destructive, but most people can judge the situation and give helpful advice.
- When I went to the meetings I listened to other people, what you should do, what you shouldn't and you get a few ideas. I didn't feel alone and made some friends.

- *I was shocked, it is always the desperate cases that come to meetings, but people shared advice and wisdom. It was really helpful for me, it took two years, but the help I got was brilliant.*
- *Women's presence at meetings often balances things out. It stops some of the men getting too anti-women and mysoginistic, this is good.*

Impact of the service

- *It took nearly three years, but I got joint custody and equal access. I don't think I could have done that without FNF.*
- *I have helped other men since that time, going to court with men as an advocate, especially for financial settlements. I have also had other Asian men contact me for help. There are more divorces within my community, and some women see the benefit system and the court as their next husband.*

This description was based on conversations with Jim Parton (current Chair), and Trevor Berry (past chair), information taken from FNF website, a visit to a Central London meeting, and conversations with three fathers.

Families Need Fathers can be contacted by writing to 134 Curtain Road, London EC2A 3AR or 0207-613-5060. FNF website address is www.fnf.org.uk.

What Works? – MAP Young Fathers' Group

Mancroft Advice Project offers information, advice and counselling to young people aged 11 to 25 in Norwich. MAP is very well established, well respected and a highly effective and professional young peoples project.

The young fathers' group was formed at the end of 1993 by two MAP volunteers, Mark Osbourne and Peter Bainbridge (both fathers). Peter later became an advice worker at MAP.

There were support groups at MAP for young mothers, for young gay men and the young fathers (who attended MAP) asked why there was no support for them as a group. They were thought (on reflection) to want their own identities acknowledged.

Initially, the group was offered to young fathers, expectant fathers or any others with an interest. The first meeting was on a Friday morning (for two hours), but later moved to a Monday evening. There were four regular attenders, who were aged from 18 to 21. Three were living at either the local YMCA or St Edmund's Hostel (and not living with their children), while the fourth was living with a partner and children. Most had been brought up in care and/or, had lost contact with their own fathers, which is thought to have contributed to the strength of their fatherhood identity.

One of the first tasks of the four fathers, was to target new members. A leaflet was produced and distributed to health centres, hostels, advice agencies and professionals working with young men.

In the last seven years, an estimated 15 young fathers have been involved, with a core of five. There have been repeated attempts to recruit more young fathers. Mark and Justin (Director of MAP) believe that personal contact is everything when trying to recruit for such a group, and while they often got referrals (especially from Social Services), having only two voluntary workers often meant that they were unable to follow these up.

From the outset, the aim was 'to provide a safe space, so that both personal and practical issues could be discussed. Some young men drifted in and out, returning when they felt the need to talk'.

Initially, the focus was on being young men (and not parenting), skills, especially negotiating and communication skills. Throughout, it has been a 'talking group'. Topics would change, with preference given to those identified by members and they have included changing relationships, families, masculinity, anger and football. Underlying all of this has been the building of the young fathers' confidence.

As the fathers dealt with a broad range of issues, those young men who were not living with their children wanted to have more contact with them, and fathering issues came to the fore. Young men were thought to be hurting when separated from their children, and this was thought to reinforce their feelings of worthlessness.

Young men's view of their own self-worth has been a recurrent theme for the majority of members; however, their commitment to the group has been very high, and without this, it would not have survived. Maintaining interest has, at times, been a struggle. Ideas have never been the problem; following them through has been a more difficult matter.

For a while, the group functioned more as a 'therapeutic group'. Although this was an uncomfortable experience for those involved, it helped the fathers to become more focused and, more respectful of each other. Youth work type worksheets were used at times to stimulate conversation and simple questions would often lead to complex discussions about families, with discussions on relationships with fathers and mothers being the most intense.

The group applied for funding from Norwich Safer Cities which was successful. The grant paid for the development of resources, a weekend residential and the production of a Young Men's Fact Pack.

As well as information on local services and facilities, a significant part of the pack related to legal issues, as many of the young fathers were ignorant of their rights (or lack of them), regarding their children. The pack also aimed to acknowledge that their situations were not unusual, and has helped them to define their roles and responsibilities as parents.

When the Pack was launched [in 1997, with 250 copies published] the media coverage was very good and the Pack was distributed throughout Norfolk. The young fathers dealt with most of the media enquiries themselves, and they 'became quite picky about who they talked to'. Two of them were asked to be on TV, with a trip to London, chauffeur driven car, hotel and posh meal out which was a new experience for them.

Justin and Mark thought that the young men were very quick to realise and understand what the media were after, and responded to them with stories that they lapped up. The media interest did cause some tensions within MAP itself. The attention given to the young fathers was resented by some other project users and even staff got fed up.

A documentary video has also been started, made by the young fathers about their situation and experiences as fathers not living with their children.

The grant changed the nature of the group; it moved from being a 'support' group to a 'work' group. Instead of talking about their lives and fatherhood, they talked about tasks that needed to be done. This suited some and made the group less desirable for others.

The main benefits that Justin and Mark thought the young fathers had gained were:

- they established or maintained contact with their children;
- they 'learnt from their mistakes', so those that have gone on to father other children have been very active from the beginning;
- that the young men shared a belief in the importance of being a good father, and while they struggled to live out that belief, the group confirmed this for them;
- they gained new skills and grew in confidence (this was particularly the case when the group was asked to be on the radio, the TV and participate in conferences). This outside recognition of their importance has

had an enormous impact on them;
- their identities as fathers were valued;
- activities such as the Fact Pack development provided an impetus for finding out a lot about the law, benefits, rights and responsibilities as well as activities and services locally.

In a write-up of the work, Peter Bainbridge said: Over the four years, I believe we have all learnt a great deal. Young men can have their feelings valued and recognised and do care for their children, even if they are unable to take part in the childcare. Our experience has shown that young men are not irresponsible, as they are often made out to be; that they feel misunderstood, not good enough and on the edge of their children's lives.

As workers, we have sometimes felt frustrated and isolated. But, in truth, these are the feelings young fathers face on a daily basis, and, until society acknowledges the importance of their role and begins to work with boys to educate them differently, they will remain.

While the Safer Cities grant brought high levels of interest in their activities, fund-raising has been very difficult. MAP and the young fathers wanted to establish a 'stand alone' service, build up their core activities (which included young fathers going into schools) and develop a team of committed volunteers, but this has not, as yet, been carried through.

What the fathers said:

The Young Fathers' Group made me more confident. I learned to listen and speak my mind. It was a bit like a family for me and helped me get my bearings and helped me grow up a lot.

If it hadn't been for Peter and the group, I think I would have been really messed up, and I did think about doing myself in.

Just talking about things helps; you have to get the hurtful bits out so you can live a bit. The group and Peter also helped me get into counselling (at MAP); I would never have done it if it wasn't for Peter, even though I really needed it.

This description of the Young Fathers' Group came from extensive conversations with Justin Rolph (Director) at MAP, and Mark Osbourne (one of the volunteer workers). Peter Bainbridge wanted to be involved, but was unable to because of family illness.

Details were also taken from Norwich Young Fathers' Group, written for Working With Men by Peter Bainbridge. Justin Rolph has written Young, Unemployed and Unmarried ... Fathers Talking (published by WWM), which is based on a series of interviews with young fathers (including those that formed the core of the Young Fathers' Group).

Man Enough

Albert Ford (who runs a leather business) was going through a divorce. He looked for help from local organisations, found himself the only man on a parenting course and felt that both help and courses were geared only towards mothers.

He attended two programmes, one with the Family Caring Trust (and their Parents' Support Group), a 15-week Family Nurturing Network (FNN) course, (which he went on to help co-facilitate). He trained to be a Parentline volunteer and became a volunteer at Ley Drug and Alcohol Centre.

Through these contacts and experience, Albert decided to develop a specific programme for fathers and with the help of Kathy Peto and the Oxford Parenting Forum, he approached the local Community Education Unit to support a fatherhood course which started in October 1998.

Being in business, Albert had some idea of the need to market the course. So leaflets about 'Man Enough' went through the Community Education magazine, Oxford Parenting Forum, libraries, through partners on other parenting courses, local schools and as fathers came into his Central Oxford shop, he gave them a leaflet and talked to them about the course. This all happened during the Summer of 1998.

Albert believes that men were attracted to the course because he stressed the importance of fathers and that the role is serious, and not to be taken lightly. He also thought that men responded to the fact that it was for fathers only.

Fifteen men registered for the first course, paying £10 for the 10-week course. Albert says that a third of the men came via personal contacts (made in his shop) and another third from personal contacts through supportive agencies.

The men themselves tended to fall into three categories: half of them were middle class men living with their partners wanting to improve their parenting skills; a quarter had teenage children that they were finding heavy going; and the other quarter were separated or stepfathers, with one granddad and one man who didn't have children, but still wanted to attend the course.

The first session saw the usual ground rules and confidentiality agreements, hopes and fears and Albert reiterating the value of fathers and fathering. The hopes and fears exercise tended to throw up issues such as:

Hopes: to learn to stop shouting at my kids;
to learn to avoid taking – or seeming to take – sides;
to be able to make being with my children more fun;
to understand how children tick;
how to be NOT my dad.

Fears: of work and other demands affecting my attendance;
of breaking confidentiality;
of realising that I am a worse dad than I thought;
of not following it all through;
of not having enough opportunities to practice and improve.

He believes that those participants with some experience of groups helped other men to talk about themselves and their lives.

Albert has been using the Family Caring Trust handbook What can a parent do? which aims to develop practical skills for those with children aged 5-15. The course has a strong emphasis on communication, and suggests that this is a key to improving discipline, co-operation and respect.

Sessions cover: discipline; becoming a responsible parent; encouragement; listening; communicating about problems and talking things through. Each session has a number of case studies focused on common problem areas (for discussion); some explanations of why children behave that way; advice and suggestions on ways to change behaviours; an exercise for participants to identify their own children's behaviour; and an expectation that something different will be tried in the week to come.

A video tape supports the handbook. Albert has found this handbook is a good basis for 'Man Enough' courses, and apart from slight changes in session titles, he has kept with the handbook format.

The two-and-a-half-hour sessions usually begin with a forum for fathers to talk about what has happened at home in the week, and how the skills they are learning have impacted.

The approach allows for a reflection on the problem, personal experience, helpful explanations and 'tips' as well as identification of the skills required and tasks for the week ahead. While Albert acknowledges that the approach does not address gender and specific issues about fathering, he believes that the practical, skills based focus of the programme works well with fathers and that it is in the discussions that fathering issues emerge. He says that most of the men find it difficult to share their personal experience, but finds that the diversity of the groups tends to help men talk.

The course relies heavily on written materials, although Albert has not found this a barrier for men with low literacy skills. He finds the hardest task during sessions is to keep the discussion focused on the session themes.

Each course is finished with a 'graduation celebration' (a clue to Albert's New York heritage) and a further 'Where do we go from here?' session.

Apart from the five courses in Oxford, at Cherwell School for the North Oxford Community Education Programme, Albert has also delivered four courses at Bullingdon Prison, at Aylesbury Young Offender Institution and another at Ley Community Drug and Alcohol Rehabilitation Centre. He has used a similar format and style, and found they have worked well.

Albert believes the course works for a number of reasons:

- the sessions tend to unpack the issues for men, allowing them to distance themselves from the difficulties, see 'what is going on', suggest various techniques and skills and encourage men to reflect rather than teach them. This allows men to feel more confident rather than inadequate;
- the course itself validates (fathers') and men's role, while most men arrive feeling as though they have lost their role or that fatherhood and even manhood are 'a bit of a mess';
- the course supports men's commitment to their children and their determination to be good fathers.

Albert clearly shares this passion and determination and obviously plays a part in making these courses work. In a recent article Albert was described as a 'Maverick', ...he is twice divorced and an ex-heroin addict. He is estranged from his two older children and is bringing up younger twin boys (shared parented). For the fathers involved in 'Man Enough', Albert's willingness to reveal such personal details is an important part of the group's success.

The five courses have averaged 15 men. Recruitment has been relatively easy, even though each course has required men to pay (with the current course costing £75, although bursaries are available). Albert has facilitated all of the courses, but has brought in two other fathers to help him. He is conscious of the courses relying heavily on him and wants to broaden 'Man Enough' to other areas.

Albert wants to develop a 'Fathers' Network' and has been experimenting with monthly open follow-up sessions.

However, because the course relies heavily on Community Education support, he has no resources to develop this. Albert has found that men do build relationships with one another during the course and want to encourage this once the course is finished. He believes that developing the Network will encourage and support this process.

Cathy Peto of FNN has known Albert since he became involved in their courses and says:

I must admit I was a bit anxious about Albert's zeal at the beginning, but I think he has learnt a lot about running groups and how to really listen to people and not pressure them with his own agenda.

He has kept his determination and this means that he is very good at following people up; he shows genuine interest and fathers know he is on their side. He also puts a huge amount of effort in preparing the room and supporting individuals.

I have always been impressed with the range of fathers attracted to the courses, affluent business men through to working class men. I think this might be because Albert is from New York and therefore groups with fathers from different classes is not such a problem; they are all able to identify with him.

What the fathers said:

About recruitment

I didn't like the way I was behaving, shouting at the kids, too tired to enjoy being with them, something had to give. I heard about the course and thought I would give it a go. When I rang Albert, he was very supportive and encouraging. I liked Albert's approach, he didn't pull any punches, but was very encouraging. It turns out I was a much better dad than I thought I was myself.

I was really nervous about going on the course, although I tried to think positive. I thought it would be formal, classroom and exam type, I would be given a test and come out a bad dad! I also thought that if I went on a course like this it would mark me out as a bad dad. After two or three weeks I came out of my shell, started to relax and talk more freely – the role plays really helped that.

I heard about the course from a mate of mine, he had done the course and said it had helped him understand his children. He knew my kids didn't live with me and I was going through a divorce and he thought the course would help.

About the course

Hearing the other men talk about things, hearing the same issues coming up in their relationships – well, you realise it's not just you that's having trouble. These are problems that fathers have, fathers in general. Paul – married man.

Being a father, it can be a very lonely place to be. I work hard, travel around a lot and often feel really tired when I go into the session – but I feel awake, really awake, when it's finished. You learn so many new things about yourself. Gordon.

He doesn't make out that he's better than us, some kind of super-perfect super-dad. He's had some horrendous experiences but has come out the other side. It's good to know that. Graham.

Talking about being a father – it's really good to have that... I was really surprised how everyone was prepared to open up quickly and discuss things that they hadn't had a chance to do before. Having that arena to talk about being a father for an hour, or a couple of hours, is really useful. Gregg.

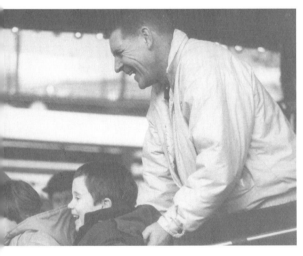

Because we are all blokes, we play a similar role, juggling work and home. The tensions we feel are similar. It was educational, we did role-plays and the practical exercises as well as become part of a group. The discussions were open and free.

The course has only just finished, but we are going to have a monthly reunion, have a topic, but feedback on our lives, keep the spark.

If it had been men and women, I think there would have been more disagreement, more upset in the group. When men say they find it difficult to make the time for their kids, there is agreement; if there were women there might be more conflict, we understood each other, I am sure it is the same when there are all women.

Albert wasn't directional, he always just suggested what we did. He was always very encouraging and understanding.

About the course's impact

There's no turning back once you start. You open up to new ideas. Once you begin, that's it. You're on that track because you made a decision to try and change and one way or another it has an effect. Paul.

My partner says she has seen me more able to be patient, I listen more, expect more from my two boys, and I am more contented.

Before the course I never knew what my kids were saying to me, I just didn't understand. About halfway through I was just ready to shout at them, when I thought 'What did the course say about this?' It gave me an awareness and insight *into what was happening. My kids say I am much better now, not shouting so much and I listen to them.*

I learnt from the group that I was normal, things I felt and thought were just normal.

This description was based on a visit and conversation with Albert Ford, reading a number of local and national articles written about him and the programme, conversations with participating fathers and Cathy Peto at the Family Nurturing Network.

1 Man Enough, September 2000, Hopes and Fears.

2 Man Enough, Oxford article on 4th January 1999.

What Can a Parent Do? (Practical skills to help parents be more responsible and effective). Michael and Terri Quinn, Family Caring Trust, 1986 available from FCT, 44 Rathfriland Road, Newry, Co. Down, BT34 1LD.

'Man Enough', can be contacted at 1 Fogwell Road, Botley, Oxford, OX2 9ZA. Tel. No: 01865-863539 or fax: 01865-862418.

What Works? – Men United

Men United started in 1994. Ron Russell was a single father caring for his 6-month-old baby; he was separated from his wider family and getting his main support from Garden Street Family Centre, in Radford. He was the only regular male user and wanted to meet with other fathers.

Ron says: *I am a single parent. I was looking after a six month old boy. I had lost all of my male friends because they did not think or believe a man should be looking after a child on his own and because I did not go out boozing and clubbing with them. I felt I was all on my own and isolated.*

Then when my son was 15 months I got him a place in the nursery at my local family centre – after a time I realised not one man visited the family centre! At a Parents' Committee meeting I decided to have a say and what I said was: 'What about a men's group?'

I tried to get men involved, but no luck. Then by some fluke there came a student social worker who decided to help me with the men's group and in no time we had three other members. At last I was not alone any more – I knew that at least once a week I could meet with them and talk to men about being a father and what its like being a father. I thought there must be other men in the same situation as me, who think like me. It took a time – but I always thought they would come.

With the support of Derek McIntosh (a social work student on placement at Garden Street), he made contact with other fathers (Centre contacts, leaflets to other projects) and a small group began to meet on a Friday morning on a drop-in basis. It started very slowly, and grew to a core of 6 fathers after a year and a half. Most were single parents and those that regularly used the drop-in came to talk to others in a similar position as themselves. They were both black and white men reflecting the community in Radford. Support, friendship and isolation were the recurrent themes voiced.

Derek left the Centre after three months and Zbyszek Luczynski (Community Worker employed by Nottinghamshire Social Services) took up the support work, but always with a strong community development approach, which included 'encouraging self-determination, the sharing of power, and the development of knowledge'.

In a leaflet produced shortly after the

group began, the members describe it as for:

all men who have children and men without children, with or without partners, to share their experience of being a man and being a father, talking about everyday things.

The drop-in continued, and then a 10 session fathers' course was planned. The focus of this course was personal experience of fathering, relationships with children, anger management and discipline. The core of 6 attended this course and others.

Referrals came from other Centre users and local social workers (especially looking to refer men who had difficulties with disciplining their children). There was a strategy of home visiting introduced. Referred men were visited by Zbyszek and one of the fathers, which usually made it easier for the fathers to access the group.

Other courses followed, such as Men's Health (with a women's health promotion worker), and a variety of sports sessions. The group have cooked together, and had infrequent meetings with the Centre's women's group to discuss common issues about parenting. They have formed a committee, got funding from the County Council, given presentations to local councillors and workshops at conferences.

Over the years an estimated 60 fathers have attended the different activities.

Most fathers have attended for a while and moved on, while 6 to 8 have been involved regularly for the last 5 years or so.

Zbyszek is of the view that men have moved on for a number of reasons:

- some men were only interested in specific initiatives;
- some men's lives were chaotic and they had difficulties sustaining their involvement;
- some just didn't get on (Zbyszek talked about one man who was racist and the other fathers found this unacceptable);
- the group also challenged other fathers' attitudes and behaviours and Zbyszek says that some of these fathers didn't like that.

Once the drop-in was established, the fathers developed their own aims, which included:

For the group to:

- encourage fathers and men to help each other;
- provide time and space to share feelings with other men;
- build a network of fathers' support groups and services for families;
- provide information and training on men's health, legal and welfare rights, parenting skills, job and careers opportunities, communication, confidence and assertion skills.

For the wider community to:

- publicise the benefits of men taking responsibility for supporting each other and their families;
- break down barriers and destroy stereotypes of how men should be;
- build a better understanding of men, women, our children and of different cultures.

(taken from a leaflet prepared by the men to advertise the group)

The focus of many of the activities has been broader than being fathers, but the core group have continued to have fatherhood at the centre of their identities. They feel particularly strongly that professionals do not take them seriously or recognise them as good parents, and that as unmarried fathers their lack of rights is at the core of what they want to see changed.

Zbyszek's role has changed as the project has developed. Initially his role was to organise speakers and help recruit fathers. He had 6 to 8 hours allocated to this aspect of his job, but tended to do much more (especially because of the home visiting).

As the group developed, and organised courses and speakers, small grants had to be applied for and handled. The group had to move towards being able to deal with finances and fund-raising. Initially, funds were raised through regular boot sales, but later small grants came from the County Council and a committee had to be formed and organised.

Zbyszek handed over certain responsibilities to members of the group and has continued his role inspite of changing his job in July 1998 (when his post was scrapped by the County Council).

His role was seen as very important by the fathers:

People like Zbyszek know things we don't; he knows the ropes, the contacts, knows who we need to know – which strings to pull. We learn these things from him. We know about looking after the children and being single dads, but not about those other things we need if this group is going to get anywhere.

He gives us information and it is up to us what we do with it. It is not his job or his place to go out and do things.

Zbyszek believes the work has a number of strengths:

- men have gained experience and got a sense of their self worth;
- they have learnt from organising the group themselves, giving presentations and from such courses as Men's Health and Anger Management;
- they have shared their experiences and supported each other in obtaining parental responsibility for their children;

- the core group has gained status (they have liked meeting people, and becoming a focus on the national stage and at conferences);
- it has empowered a number of fathers to take on organising the group;
- they have taken on professionals;
- they have learnt parenting skills;
- and stood up for themselves.

Some of the men felt they had gained personally. Some have gone on college courses and some found jobs, including one man who became a mid-day supervisor at a local school (certainly one of the first in Nottingham). One man had cut down on his smoking as a result of the health education sessions.

More recently, it has been difficult to keep the group going. Zbyszek's post (and those of other Community Development workers), has been cut by the Council, and when they knew he was leaving, the group decided they wanted to apply for funding to set up a Centre and have a full-time worker of their own.

The Council allocated a female community worker to the group. The fathers met with her, set some ground rules (she couldn't attend their meetings) and the fathers say she was very helpful, but this arrangement only lasted for six months; her post was also cut by the Council.

Zbyszek says that the group have become anti-professional, and disappointed that he wasn't doing enough personally. This has led to the men feeling as though the authorities have let them down. 'They have become disillusioned, been knocked back and turned bitter,' says Zbyszek, and no local professionals are willing to support them (i.e. no one is willing to be a Trustee). Zbyszek is of the view that these working class fathers need the support of middle class fathers to legitimise the organisation.

Before Zbyszek left, the group received a grant from The Lottery (for £5,000), to carry out a 'needs assessment of local fathers' and produce a video to provide evidence for their application for a grant to set-up a Centre and employ a worker. Robert Dutton (one of the very active fathers) says: We are working with both the Nottingham and Trent Universities and have about 50 hours of video tape. This only needs to be edited now and the research is almost finished as well.

What the fathers said:
Recruitment

A mate of mine went there. I felt bored and a bit depressed, but not that bored. I thought they would be a load of bible bashers. I had been to Gingerbread, but they didn't want men there. He kept saying 'come on let's go there' and one day I did go. I wasn't the only single father, there were others going through what I was. I felt better after one meeting and kept going.

When I went to the Family Centre, there

were some women who were breast-feeding and others who had been battered by men; they didn't want men around.

A lad I knew was part of the group. I didn't need to go. When I was going through the court about my kids, there wasn't any help, so I wanted to go to see what I could do for other lads.

I didn't really go for anything, it was out of curiosity, it appealed to me. I thought something needed to be done for fathers.

What was on offer

I really enjoyed the Men's Health course, learnt about what to eat, what to feed the kids, about testicular cancer, and sex education for the kids, what to tell them and when.

It worked because we was all blokes together.

We had a computer course; they came to us, we didn't have to go to the college.

I found the anger management and facilitating course really useful.

Impact of the programme

I didnt want to become secretary of the group, my reading and writing was atrocious. I skived off school, but it made me learn.

It was something I was always looking for. I mean every bloke in this room was in the same boat as me. They was all single fathers, they have all had the same hassle as

I had. I knew what he had been through and he knew what I was going through. It wasn't what I had expected – but at the same time it was what I needed.

My partner abused my kids – not sexually, but physically and mentally abused them – I was cracking up. The good thing about the group is you can tell these and they ain't going to laugh – if you go to the pub with your mates they'd laugh, but there he has been through the same stuff and so has he and him too – he ain't going to laugh. It didn't matter what problem you come with, they will take it serious.

I have also learnt a lot about my health, for example testicular cancer, that is just one thing I should know about, but didn't. Where can a man go to ask these things? With his Doctor? I don't think so, too embarrassed to go. But when you are in a men's club, this is one thing we can talk about openly, plus it is one thing that is not talked about in the pub!

We are happy for women to come to the group when there is a purpose to it – like the health visitor, the solicitor. We wouldn't want to be seen as anti-women; It is just there are some things it is easier to talk about as men.

When we went to talk to those councillors we was all dead nervous, that was scary. But we did it and we were pleased with ourselves. They said they were impressed with what we were doing and that.

The men in this group challenge the stereotype of fathers being involved in the care of their children. They also challenge the stereotype that men can't, won't and don't share emotions, feelings, anxieties and hopes with each other.

It (the group) has really brought me out of myself. I was a bit shy before, but as I have gone to court with lads and to Social Services' case conferences, I have had to speak my mind and sometimes talk harsh with the guys.

This description was based on conversations with Zbyszek Luczynski and five fathers. Also, various write-ups of the work including Men United (fathers' voices) by Jennie Fleming and Zbyszek Luczynski in Groupwork, vol 11, No 2, 1999. pages 21-37 and the description in Fathers Figure: fathers' groups in family policy by Emma Longstaff. IPPR, London 2000.

Men United can be contacted via: Robert Dutton, 3 Huggett Gardens, Top Valley, Nottingham, NG5 9ER.

What works? NEWPIN Fathers' Project

NEWPIN is a national voluntary organisation, set up in 1980, which helps parents under stress break the cyclical effects of destructive family behaviour. Through a network of 16 local centres, NEWPIN aims to provide long-term emotional support to enable both parents and children to develop their full potential. Each centre offers a home visiting and befriending scheme, family play, groupwork, counselling and personal development programmes.

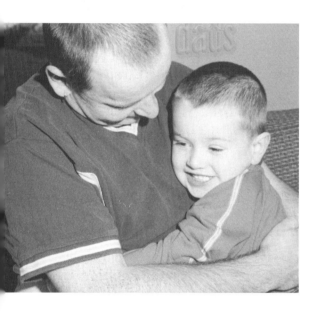

The origins of the fathers' project were in 1994, when it was recognised that *'lack of support for men to develop positive, close relations with their children was a major social problem with damaging consequences for the whole family.* An 18 week pilot project was devised by Ann Jenkins-Hansen (NEWPIN's then Clinical Director) working with an outside psychotherapist (Paul Wolf-Light), who worked at a local Domestic Violence programme for men.

This pilot was attended by partners of mothers using NEWPIN services in South London, and this led to the appointment of a consultant (for one day a week), in October 1996 (David Bartlett), which was funded by a local Charitable Trust.

The first programme was started in September 1997, so 11 months were spent establishing the project and recruiting fathers. There were a number of mailings to agencies. Numerous social workers' team meetings were visited; there were discussions with Social Services managers, health visitors, court welfare officers, drug and alcohol project workers and probation services. They were often enthusiastic about the establishment of a fathers' programme.

However, referrals were very slow in coming through, for a number of reasons. They included agencies being enthusiastic, but having little contact with fathers; some having low expectations of the men they were working with; others such as Probation, who were looking for short-term programmes to help deal with men's violence and anger; and still others being enthusiastic, but just not getting around to referring fathers.

The 'low expectations' took the form both of a low view of men's parenting potential, and a low expectation that they would use any service. For some agencies, it was just not a priority – i.e. they saw fathers as peripheral to family life, and working with or referring them would have been seen as a very low priority.

David also thought that there were some organisations 'who DID see it as a priority, but did not want to refer to us' – they wanted to work with them themselves! This is only a hunch, and only applies to a couple of agencies in the voluntary family support field.

Some agencies misconstrued what we were about; despite clear statements that we were for all fathers, they thought we were for non-resident and/or single fathers. They seemed to find it hard to imagine fathers living with the mother of the children had any support needs. (I think this was a significant conceptual hurdle for agencies to overcome before they could begin to refer.)

David says: The referring agency that changed its behaviour most was definitely social services. This reflected my going to meetings more, so that by the referral-to-second-group stage, our reputation improved. I suspect, even though I had the NEWPIN name behind me, some agencies/workers were suspicious of my motives. Was I a fathers' rights' group? Was I really focusing enough on the child's interests? Certainly, they slowly changed their view about the importance of working with fathers.

On reflection, David believes that while the visits were labour intensive, they were much more effective than the written dissemination, and that they often found themselves concentrating on agencies that produced very little, while the referring agencies were often the ones that saw a lot of men, and had a pool to refer from.

David says: Some people think dads will only come to groups with a strongly practical focus. Our mailings did not strongly emphasise practical activities or outcomes – I felt that the important point was to talk about the group belonging in some sense to the dads, and that it was there because dads were important. I also talked about overcoming isolation, as well as organising activities.

One of the difficulties of the programme,

was that it was 35 weekly (two-and-a-half hour) sessions, so a long commitment for men whose lives were often a little chaotic. However, there were 32 referrals to the first programme, the bulk of which came from social services, voluntary sector agencies, and solicitors.

Half dropped out before they were interviewed. Five dropped out post interview, four of them single fathers – two of whom said they could not find anyone to undertake childcare for the weekday evening of the group. Therefore there were 10 men who started the first programme which dropped to seven in the second week.

The initial interviews suggested that fathers were wary of services for families, and did not expect them to be supportive to fathers. The project had to work hard to establish trust by giving a clear message that the group would be a place where their experiences, feelings and aspirations as fathers would be taken seriously.

A number of factors stood out as common to the seven fathers who started the programme:

● they had had prior experience of therapeutic work (i.e. in drug rehabilitation);
● none of the fathers lived in nuclear families (two parents with their genetic offspring). Of the five resident fathers, two were living in 'reconstituted' families with both

genetic and stepchildren, and the other three were lone parents;
● there was a strong thread of both parents having difficulties that made it hard for them to parent effectively. Of the six living mothers, five had patterns of chronic alcohol/drug abuse or moderate/serious mental health problems;
● nearly all of the men were feeling depressed, or severely depressed at interview, and one had a long-term manic depressive condition. Four of the men had had severe drug/alcohol problems in the past and five reported serious childhood physical abuse from their fathers, and the other two had fathers with serious alcohol problems;
● ages ranged from 34-47 years and ethnically there were four white British, one Italian, one Jewish and one Turkish Cypriot.

The aims of the programme were to give men a greater understanding of (and support in) their role as carers of children, so they could make permanent improvements in family relationships.

The broad objectives were to:

● enhance fathers' understanding of the developmental/emotional needs of children, and for them to develop specific skills and knowledge that foster competent and nurturing parenting;
● do this within a reflective and supportive framework that addressed

attitudes, psychological and cultural issues that shape individual fathers' parenting and family relationships.

The programme was co-facilitated by Barbara Plows (a full-time worker with NEWPIN, and an experienced group worker) and David Bartlett.

David says:

Barbara and I spent a lot of time in advance discussing our feelings and attitudes about fatherhood and masculinity and working in a group. By the time the group started, we knew each other quite well, and trusted each other. Above all, this helped us to provide a safe space for the men, and a model of how a man and a woman can negotiate and co-operate effectively.

They trusted us to work well together. Some of the men felt less comfortable with a woman at first because of their own poor relationships with women. Others found it harder to open up with me because they still felt scared of their fathers' abusiveness and authoritarianism. But these projections about the men's mothers and fathers were worked on within the group.

Each session was divided into educational and therapeutic slots. The educational section covered such issues as masculine identity; what is a father?; relationships with mothers and fathers; aggression and violence; communication and problem-solving with adult partners and children's psychological and physical needs. In addition to the weekly sessions, there were also an additional three meetings (at weekends), with fathers and children for lunch and play activities.

The workers believed that the men liked the structure that a weekly discussion topic provided, and were not put off by the personal nature of the subjects. This was illustrated by the goals that men themselves identified for the group at the outset, which included:

● sharing experiences and feeling less alone;
● gaining confidence as a parent;
● exploring the impact of their upbringing on their parenting;
● learning to look after themselves and not having unrealistic expectations of themselves as fathers;
● understanding their children better;
● learning how to control angry feelings, and getting advice on how to handle specific difficult situations.

The 'therapeutic' slot was less structured, where the men could explore their feelings in more depth, both about the discussion topic and other issues of importance to them. In practice, there was a lot of overlap, and the facilitators did not hold the group rigidly to the agenda, if something was thought to be more important. The facilitators were surprised by how quickly the group discussions took off, believing that the fathers quickly felt that it was a non-judgemental and supportive setting.

David says:

Group discussions took off because it was seen as supportive – but that was both about the 'setting', and about the realisation that there was a common experience and purpose that the men shared (so what we did as facilitators was partly to help the dads realise that there was common ground).

Often there didn't feel to be enough time, and it was hard to give enough space to both the 'structured/educational' and 'therapeutic' elements of the programme. Several of the men expressed a desire for two sessions a week.

From the discussion at the end of the course, most of the men said that the course had had a major impact on their relationship with their children.

Most of them had learnt different ways of relating to their children (shouting and hitting less, remaining calmer, listening more).

They reported that they were less bound up in feelings of anger and shame, were more confident, more open with their feelings, and were aware of their children's needs.

They also built supportive relationships with other fathers outside the group (usually via the phone), but this took a long time to develop.

Since this initial programme (that ended in April 1998), the project has developed substantially. There is now a separate Fathers' Centre (based in a Sure Start area), with two full-time workers, and the programme now has two formats, an eight-week as well as the nine-month programme. There have been a further five groups, and more than 40 men have now attended. There are usually 6 or 7 fathers starting and most stay for the duration.

A number of significant changes have occurred in the last two-and-a-half years:

a) Referrals are now mainly word of mouth, and from agencies that have referred men before and seen them change. In addition, men have more recently come from the Project's outreach work (in the street, supermarkets, fairs, community events and train stations) and current workers have found the separate centre has helped in recruiting men. Interestingly, they have found that the less preparation men have for the sessions, the more likely they are to come.

David says: *The long phone call can do one of two things – (1) indicate that the person is not ready for a group, or has issues that don't fit (so that is why the call is long – to resolve issues on the phone, as they won't be coming in – e.g. someone who wants advice about splitting up, and a bit of support, but doesn't want to attend any groups); or (2) show that the call brought up feelings that they didn't feel safe with. So NEWPIN tends to offer dads enough to get them to come in – but not too much.*

b) The profile of the fathers has also changed. While the age range has broadened slightly (now 25 to 40), there are men who are wanting to be with other fathers and actively improve their fathering. More non-resident fathers are attending, mainly as a result of their lack of contact with their children and some a desire for the contact that has been agreed by the courts. A number of men are now requesting advice on contact and related issues.

c) The programme continues to be delivered by two facilitators, but these have changed, with programmes being delivered by two men, a man and a woman, a black man and white man, and a black man and white woman. Interestingly, when a black facilitator has been involved, black men have come forward for the programme, most of whom were in mixed relationships (reflecting the local community).

d) The workers are of a view that it was easier to deal with issues about (heterosexual) sex, when a female facilitator was not there, while it was easier to talk about men's friendships when a woman was there. Issues about race and culture issues were driven by the presence of black men. However, there was also a view that issues raised during the different programmes were much the same, while issues emerged earlier or later, in part, dependent on the profile of the co-facilitators. This was seen as one of the benefits of such a long programme as most issues eventually emerged.

e) As the fathers' programme (and more recently Fathers' Centre) has become more established, tensions are thought to have emerged within NEWPIN. Core activities have always been with women and children and often involved child protection and domestic violence issues. Concerns about women's safety have been raised, as have views that the work with fathers has grown too big and/or too independent of NEWPIN.

Senior management's commitment to fathers' work was thought to have been influential in protecting these developments. There was also a view that when fathers had become involved in activities (within NEWPIN) with mothers, their shared experience (especially of isolation and depression), overcame gender differences. Other NEWPIN centres have also shown an interest in the fathers' work.

f) Originally, funding came from a local charitable trust (for the pilot and also the consultant), and now comes through the Home Office Family Support Unit for 1999-2002, to extend the programme in South London.

g) Longer-term funding has enabled the project to begin to devise specific programmes for black fathers, young fathers, non-resident fathers, and fathers involved in the criminal justice or court welfare systems. The original nine-month format has provided a very useful foundation for designing and implementing these focused support services. Comments from internal evaluations, and feedback from local community groups suggest that a shorter course made available at regular intervals would attract more fathers, but the demand for longer courses remains.

While each of the programmes has been recorded by the facilitators, and fathers were asked at the end to comment and reflect on the value to them, there has been no external evaluation.

What fathers said:

I was getting counselling from an alcohol clinic, I had just been divorced and I was hoping it would be a source of support and they would help fathers under stress.

I met David (the worker) and I got the impression it would be worth a whirl.

I realised I was not alone, that there were other blokes in a similar position, and it helped me to turn bad experiences into good use.

I learnt a lot listening to other guys, about the CSA, about looking after kids and about being a better parent.

To contact NEWPIN Fathers' Support Programme phone Celestine Chakravarty-Agbo (centre manager) 0207 740 8997, or write to The Fathers' Centre, The Amersham Centre, Inville Road, London SE17 2HY.

This description of NEWPIN's fathers' work was written after a meeting with Celestine Chakravarty-Agbo and David Bartlett, phone conversations with two fathers and reading various articles and write-ups of the work.

What Works? – Pen Green Family Centre

Pen Green Family Centre for under-fives and their families opened in 1983 and is jointly funded by social services and the LEA. The aim of the Centre is to offer a comprehensive service for parents and their children in a friendly and stimulating environment by providing: community-based day care nursery with education for 60 children; and family support services through nursery provision, community adult education programmes, health resources and family work.
The services have grown and developed over the years and are very much needs-led by the families that use the Centre.

This piece of fathers' work will be described in a wider context than most others in this report, because Pen Green have approached work with fathers as part of a wider gender strategy and to describe the fathers' group in isolation from the rest would be selling it short; but first the fathers' group.

Initiated by Trevor Chandler, the need for a fathers' group came about because staff acknowledged that:

● fathers were an important part of the family and, if fathers were to be involved, a number of strategies would be needed;

● men can feel isolated and de-skilled as parents;

● several men who use the Centre had expressed the interest to meet and wanted to attend activities, but felt intimidated by predominantly female groups.

Started in 1988, the men's group was advertised within the Centre, and through other professionals (especially in health and social services). Probation were also mailed, and wanted to refer men who were violent. These referrals were thought to be inappropriate, as they required a more specialist service.

The first evening there was only one man; the second evening there were two, and within two months there were eight participants. Trevor is of the view that there was a 'buzz' about the group and this brought men out eventually. They met for two hours a week on a Thursday evening with the aims of:

● providing somewhere for men to talk about their personal feelings and share their hopes and fears as parents and as partners;

- raising gender awareness and taking personal responsibility for how men respond and relate to each other, to women and to children;
- exploring issues around being a man and male identity, and overcoming internal and external stereotypes;
- providing a forum within which to develop trusting relationships and overcome feelings of isolation.

Men came from diverse backgrounds and had different expectations of the group. They were aged 25 years upwards, most with young children and from a broad range of professional, manual, employed, self-employed and unemployed categories.

A number of issues emerged early on; these included guilt for some men about the number of hours they worked, and regrets they had about not spending time with their children. There was a split within the group between those interested in being much more personal (which included both reflections on their own experience and also the development of skills, such as dealing with conflict situations), and others who wanted to look at the politics of gender (focusing on the justice system, child abuse and inequalities in the workplace and home).

Trevor says it wasn't an easy group to lead, in spite of his extensive experience of training and groupwork:

I was trapped by my own fear and fantasies of being in an all-male group, and, in the process, de-skilled myself. As a consequence, the group got off to a slow faltering start: group members generally were tentative in our interactions and unclear about what we were there for and how we wanted to use our time together.

Different ways of structuring were tried: planned subjects (such as fatherhood, sexuality and violence); and a more open structure where men could bring issues. Trevor says that over the first 18 months the meetings were varied in terms of how satisfying they were for participants.

In was decided (by Trevor and a consultant in groupwork), that it was important that the group became either a personal development group or one that looked at the politics of gender: personal development became the primary focus. Some men left as they found the approach too risky, and as new members joined, the level of risk taking increased.

The weekly sessions were interspersed with activity days away and also a weekend; these helped to build trust and enabled men to be more open with one another.

All of the men's group members were also involved in delivering a 10-week programme (attended by another seven men), initiated by the local adult education institute. This was a discussion-based course where the content included sessions on 'feelings – boys don't cry' and 'masculinity – what does it mean?'

The group were also involved in a day's meeting with the Centre's women's group and while Trevor was concerned that it may be 'World War 3', the day showed that the men and women often had the same aspirations, but talked about them and dealt with them differently. Trevor was of the view that a common humanity emerged that had a big impact on everyone – including staff.

The men's group went on for 10 years, stopping in 1998. While this was always a men's group (and not just about fatherhood), it represents only a small part of the gender-based work carried out at Pen Green. Probably the most significant (and unusual) aspect of this work is that gender has become explicit for staff, parents and the children.

Trevor says that when the group was started, he took confidentiality very seriously and said very little about what happened. This led to a number of fantasies from both staff and mothers about what went on. The two most common were that they brought in beer and talked about football or that they spent their time 'slagging off women'.

These stereotypes could have gone on unquestioned; however, events such as the men's and women's groups meeting for the day helped to challenge some deep seated attitudes.

Staff awareness and skills in this area were seen as very important if issues of gender were to be dealt with. Staff were asked two basic questions: 'What are we doing to enable fathers to use the Centre?' and 'What else can we do?'

This alone led to staff reviewing areas such as the physical environment and basic communication. The Centre environment was very child and mother focused, with photographs of women and children, children's painting and designs and poetry by women. It was found that this increased men's wariness.

Several fathers had commented on the difficulties they had coming into the building. They said they were not sure how to behave, who to talk to and what to say. There was no evidence of the Centre celebrating or acknowledging the role of fathers. In order to redress the balance, positive images of men were displayed.

Forms were rewritten specifically to include fathers rather than 'parents' (usually assumed to mean mothers). When writing to parents, both parents were named. On the application form for nursery places, information on both parents' working hours was asked for so that meetings could be offered at times when both parents could attend.

It was discovered that often when letters were sent to parents, they would only be read by the mother. They would sometimes not inform the father about the letter because they did not think that he would be interested. It was therefore important to arrange to talk directly with the fathers as well.

The staff spent time together in training sessions on gender issues. Nursery staff found that their expectations of fathers and male workers were to some degree influenced by what they had experienced with their own fathers. Staff found that this exploration led to staff listening more openly to fathers and they made fewer assumptions about how they saw fathers behaving with their children in nursery.

A piece of action research carried out with a small group of fathers by Angela Malcolm (a nursery nurse), raised her and other staffs' understanding of the difficulties facing local dads (most hinge around their preoccupation with the need to earn money to provide financial security for their family, and their desire to spend time with their children).

In another initiative, video cameras recorded staff greeting parents as they brought their children to the nursery. When this was analysed, staff found that there was a lot more eye contact between the staff and the mothers, and staff stood closer to mothers and sometimes made physical contact with them. Nursery staff also tended to talk and chat longer and in more depth with mothers than with fathers, with the quality of contact with fathers much less in quantity and quality.

These realisations have led to eye contact conversations and offers of support from staff to fathers. As a result, fathers are thought to stay longer in nursery and have said that they feel more comfortable bringing their children in now that they know the staff better.

The gender of the group leader is also thought to be critical. A male co-leader increases the likelihood of involving men in groups. In more therapeutic groups, Trevor says that group leaders experience strong transference and projections which are gender-based.

This increased knowledge and engagement, as well as ongoing reflection, has also led to the Centre thinking more about how they can attract fathers to events and services. Tina Bruce has been offering sessions for parents about the educational curriculum for some while now. When publicity has stressed that she is a Professor and an 'expert', and the sessions titled 'How to boost your children's brain power' fathers have attended. This approach has been used for a range of activities.

Some thought has also been given to when events and sessions are held. There is a lot of low paid, unskilled work in Corby, and it is not unusual for parents to work two shifts (6am to 2pm and 2pm to 10pm). This knowledge of family work patterns has helped staff to plan sessions to enable fathers as well as mothers to attend activities and sessions.

These activities have gone on intermittently for the last 12 years. As children have attended the nursery and other sessions, so have their parents and 87% of fathers (who have children in nursery) have become involved in sessions and activities.

Trevor would be the first to admit that gender initiatives need to be part of an integrated approach to the Centre's work with families and that there is also a need to be consistently evaluating strategies to include fathers and male carers.

There are not large numbers of fathers involved in the Centre on an ongoing basis. However, the Centre has taken on the involvement of fathers as a serious activity, and believes that there is no easy solution and that the range of initiatives have led staff to think about fathers. Those fathers who are involved are thought to feel more valued and staff question and challenge the role of fathers as parents.

What the fathers said:

Staff have always been interested in fathers' views.

Sometimes being the only father in a group is a bit of a novelty for them and nice to get the attention for me. You are constantly asked 'what's the man's view?'

I first came to a class with my wife, I think it made it easier for me. If I had been on my own, I would have had to make a lot more of an effort.

This description of the fathers' involvement work at Pen Green has been a result of a meeting with Trevor Chandler (Head of Centre), who has worked at Pen Green since 1986 and two fathers. (Since the fathers' group has finished, the Centre has lost contact with them.)

Also sections have been taken from Working With Fathers in a Family Centre (in Working With Men, 1996), Daring to Care – Men and Childcare, written by Trevor Chandler in Working with Parents edited by Margy Whalley, Hodder and Stoughton, London, 1997.

Also, other papers supplied by Pen Green Centre and a telephone conversation with one of the fathers. (Most of the other fathers involved in the initiatives described above have moved away from the Centre.)

Pen Green can be contacted by writing to Pen Green Family Centre, Pen Green Lane, Corby, Northants, NN17 1BJ or phoning 01536-400068.

What Works? – Rugby Parents' Centre

Rugby Parents' Centre is funded by the local Education Authority and has been in existence since 1983. The Centre works with a range of local agencies to offer daytime, evening and weekend programmes for parents and carers with under-fives. An estimated 400 families use the Centre's facilities, even though staffing levels are relatively low, with only two full-time workers. Parenting courses, one-to-one support and home visiting; information on education (and schools) and support for families with special needs (such as speech therapy) are all offered by the Centre. The Centre aims to offer services and courses that do not stigmatise parents or their children.

In 1994, Centre workers began to notice how few fathers used their services. Of those who did, some only came to one or two sessions, while others were either aggressive or asked for services specifically for fathers. They also found that mothers using the Centre said that their partners needed to come on courses as well. A common picture was thought to be that mothers went on parenting courses, returned home and came into conflict with their partners, because they wanted to change aspects of their parenting style. Mothers wanted their partners to attend courses, but said they were more likely to come to a specific course for fathers.

In response to this, the Centre employed David Charles-Edwards, an experienced independent management consultant (and also a father), as a course tutor to run a six, one-and-a-half-hour session course for fathers. An article appeared in the local paper, a leaflet was produced and distributed to families using the Centre and through other local agencies.

Eight fathers registered for the first course, with recruitment being relatively easy. The fathers either came as a response to the local paper article, or were partners of women who used the Centre. The course attracted a mixture of fathers: some had had experience of therapeutic activities, these were often professional, while others were much less familiar with this type of course. All of the fathers who attended the initial (and following) courses were living with their children and with a partner.

Fathers' ages ranged from 20s to 50s, and their children from new borns to teenagers.

The course was offered as an opportunity for fathers who wished to increase their understanding and strengthen their skills of fathering. The main focus of the course was on fathering and family life (sessions included 'being a father', 'fathers and sons (and gender issues)' and 'freedom, control and discipline'), although more general discussions about being a man were also commonplace.

The format was usually a short input (by David) or some kind of exercise to stimulate thought or experience, followed by a discussion and personal reflection on the session theme. Fairly traditional groupwork methods were used (group discussion, with pairs to reflect and explore personal experience), with any skills development being coincidental.

The course worked on the basis of personal experience and discussion leading to reflection, that in turn would lead to participants developing their parenting skills. This method would impact on family relationships, by 'helping men become better fathers by providing a safe and secure environment in which they could explore their feelings and experience around the role of fathers'. David is of the view that the course also provided participants with support within their fathering role and as men.

What constituted good parenting was discussed, although David says that they 'encouraged men to work it out for themselves?' However, when asked, David's list was the same as it would have been for what is a good mother. Consistent, honest, clear boundaries, listening and not always being right were all there.

Five other courses followed this initial one, usually averaging 7 fathers, so more than 40 fathers to date have been on a course at the Centre. The 6 session format has been retained, and further funding has been received from Warwickshire Health Trust and through the Community Safety Fund.

The courses have continued to be run by a tutor (although David was joined by Terry McDermott, a psychotherapist, and then Terry carried on when David took on another job), but the focus has sometimes been more therapeutic in nature mainly determined by the course tutor. Sessions have reflected this, with stronger emphasis on personal experiences. Each course has started with an initial session where men can decide whether it is for them. This is thought to have helped enable men to make up their minds at the beginning, rather than in the middle of the course.

While the format of the sessions has also remained the same, participants have either requested or suggested a range of other ways of meeting: some men wanted to meet in the pub (to make the sessions more social); some favoured going with and some without their children.

As a response to this, Saturday morning fun sessions (for under 5's) operated at the Centre for 6 months. Partners were thought to be supportive of this, primarily because it gave them a break. On average, 13 dads attended these sessions. Popular enough; however, the sessions were run by a volunteer (David), who had his 5 children with him, which made anything other than providing the environment difficult.

While the first course was relatively easy to recruit fathers for, as the courses have gone on, it has become increasingly difficult. Word-of-mouth and the partners of current Centre users have continued to be the main source of recruitment, but these have slowed down.

The courses stopped in 1998, primarily because recruitment had dried up (David and Terry having new commitments) and there was still no male worker employed to help promote the project and recruit new group members. The Centre had exhausted its own user families, but had not built up the momentum to generate recruits from outside. Unemployment rates are relatively low in Rugby; however, many of the jobs have low pay and it is not unusual for men to have 2 or 3 part-time jobs.

Violence and discipline have been common themes of the courses, but also one of the main recruitment elements. Fathers have mentioned having difficulties with anger and their children, and their partners suggesting the course as a way to deal with their tempers.

Each course has ended with all of the fathers (with their children) going for a picnic, with plenty of football and cricket. While the fathers and children have enjoyed these, they were the only sessions that were thought to have raised concerns for mothers. There was a view that this may have been because they thought that fathers were not really competent enough to look after their children or that 'mothers were threatened' that fathers could, in fact, look after them.

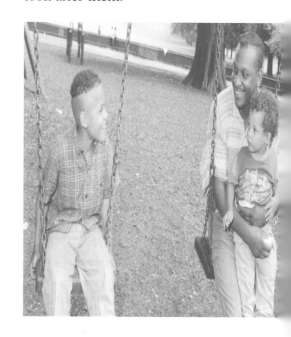

There is a substantial Black and minority ethnic community in Rugby, but there has only been 1 non-white father attending the courses. He was an Asian man referred by Social Services, who valued the course content, and also because it was a course outside of his community. Again this was put down to the non-stigmatising approach used by the Centre.

While the Centre views these courses as a success, they have not led to a substantial increase in the number of men getting involved in other services. A small proportion of men attend non-gendered courses, but hardly any come to the drop-in or specific support services.

Although courses have stopped, interest in fathers' work is still strong. An application was made to fund a 'Fathers' Network', which aimed to take the learning and experience of the fathers' groups wider and promote the importance of fathering in Rugby. More regular courses, training for professional workers and an informal support network for fathers were some of the main objectives. However, this application failed.

The Centre's view at the moment is that developments in the near future need to concentrate on new fathers ('catch men when they are motivated') and with young men who are not as yet fathers.

Four fathers were spoken to about the courses that they attended. Below are some of the comments that emerged from these conversations:

In response to the question: 'Why did you attend the course?' one man said: *My wife gave me a nudge, I suppose I went to the course to make her happy. She said that if I didn't like it I could always stop going, that helped. Also, I am not from this area, and my work means that I don't meet a lot of people, so I saw this as an opportunity to meet a few people. My wife's attitude did change, later in the course, she would say: 'Oh, so you're to see your queer fellows'.*

For all the fathers talked to, it was their wives who had been involved in the Centre's activities who had introduced them or encouraged them to go. *My wife said I needed to sort out getting angry with the children. I did have a short temper and I didn't like getting angry.*

Another said: *I was having problems with my eldest lad, he was a bit hyperactive, and his behaviour was really getting us down. My wife had been on a positive parenting course and I thought I would go. I didn't need much persuading, anyway, I'm game for anything.*

And another: *My wife mentioned it, she always goes (to the Centre) with the kids. I was having trouble with my son, losing my temper, didn't know how to deal with him.*

Fathers' views of the course were also very similar:

It gave me ideas about how to deal with my

son. I don't lose my temper any more and I learnt how to communicate with him.

I realised I was jealous of my son, he was getting all the attention. The course helped me deal with that and I don't shout at him any more.

The course gave me loads of ideas, made me realise how negative I was thinking about me son. Other fathers were in a similar position, that helped, and we all just chipped in with ideas.

I got to know a lot of blokes, one I have become friendly with. People were really committed; we had a consistent turn out.

Talking with other fathers and finding that we have the same problems was very helpful.

My wife and I seem at last to be on the same side when it comes to discipline: it used to cause a lot of arguments between us than it does now.

I'm spending more times with the kids than I was.

I realise that I've got more choices than I thought I had in the kind of dad I am.

I've learned how to control my aggression better.

Although he is an old man now, the course helped me sort out a few things with my own dad: we're better friends as a result.

No formal evaluation of any of the courses has taken place. This description was compiled after discussions with Liz Dodds (Head of Rugby Parents' Centre), David Charles-Edwards (course leader) and four fathers who attended at least one of the courses.

The courses have also produced a Fathers' Course Training Manual written by Ian Macwhinnie in association with David Charles-Edwards and Terry MacDermott which is available from the Rugby Parents' Centre, Claremont Road, Rugby CV21 3LU. 01788-579488. This Manual describes the range of sessions used within the courses and offers guidelines for trainers.

What Works? – West Wiltshire Family Centre

The West Wiltshire Family Centre in Trowbridge is a Barnardos projects which opened in 1996. The Family Centre provides a range of centre-based and outreach services to families with children in need and under 11, who live in the West Wiltshire area.
They provide a resource that aims to meet the needs of families experiencing difficulties for a broad variety of reasons – personal issues, family relationships, their physical and social environment or their financial situation.
They also aim to provide services that are open, non-stigmatising and flexible enough to respond to families in their many forms, dimensions and with their individual and personal histories.

This description of the work of West Wiltshire Family Centre concentrates on their fathers' groups and father and sons' groups. While this work started in 1999, Colin Holt (a part-time senior practitioner), who was the lead worker on these groups, has been developing work with fathers for some years within Barnardos, in Bristol. This write-up attempts to capture some of that experience as well.

Colin believes there are six good reasons for working with fathers within a family centre setting:

- *Many men are often very isolated and need an environment where they can share and explore fathering skills with other fathers.*

- *Many fathers have not received basic information on child care, child development and health issues, often given to mothers through education, health centres and life experience.*

- *Fathers who are primary carers need a supportive and educative setting which views fathers as equally competent parents as mothers.*

- *Fathers find most child-focused agencies are mother-focused and therefore they feel excluded or isolated.*

- *Many children under five years have little or no experience of other men except their own father. The Centre through group work provides a positive caring image of men.*

● *Fathers often feel excluded from Social Services Department intervention. Fathers need to have a voice within child protection investigations.*

There have been two fathers' discussion groups jointly run by West Wilts Family Centre and the Trowbridge Resource Centre (which is part of the Social Services Department). Both agencies had been trying to involve fathers (especially through drop-ins and couple work), and identified 15 fathers currently living with families, who they thought would respond to the first fathers' group.

They also sent adverts to local agencies, which generated a further 4 referrals. Colin says that when they visited these fathers, they 'were the dads from hell'; they were all violent and they were men that the referring agencies were unable to engage with, let alone work with.

Colin's previous experience had led him to expect very few referrals from outside agencies. He says that agencies are reluctant to refer to new groups; only really wanted to refer men they could not work with themselves or were viewed as difficult. They are not usually knowledgeable enough about the group or in engaging fathers to refer appropriately.

He has also found that information doesn't often get to the right workers; and, of course, another problem has been that a number of potential referral agents have very limited contact with fathers themselves. This increases the possibilities of inappropriate referral.

Colin had a lot to say about recruitment and the referral process. He said that at West Wilts they have organised dinner time seminars for agencies wanting to involve fathers, and while attendance was good (mostly health visitors, for example), he found if he talked about the work too broadly, they would switch off and usually only really engaged when they had a father to refer. He has also often found that agencies don't always know a lot about the fathers, and are too often eager to refer without really engaging with them.

Letters were sent to all the men and they were visited by both Colin and Ian Tustin. They have found that this way the men hear about the group accurately and that they can sell the aspects they think the men will respond to:

● fathers can contribute and not just receive;
● they will be fully involved and 'not be done to';
● they will build on the fathers' strengths and see them as competent.

Colin has found that this supports fathers to get involved and make best use of the opportunities the groups provide. He has also found that men are more likely to get to the first session, because they have met the two workers involved.

For the second group, flyers were sent to social services fieldwork teams, health centres, junior and infants schools, local community psychiatric services and the educational welfare services. Six referrals came from Social Services, 6 from the Resource Centre, 5 from the Family Centre and 3 from the schools. All 20 were contacted, with 8 fathers visited, 6 written to and 6 phoned. Six fathers attended the group, 2 of these had been visited and 4 had been contacted by phone.

The group was discussion-based, with each session starting off with information from the group leaders and other invited guests on the chosen topic, followed by a discussion. Fathers were asked what topics they wanted to cover, and these themes included boundaries, discipline, children's needs as they get older, challenging behaviour, fathers' and mothers' roles and step-parenting. Theses themes made up most of the group's 11 sessions.

While the group was made up of fathers with children under 5 to teenagers; those with experience of structured group work and those with none; long-term unemployed and those working and primary carers and step-fathers, these differences were not thought to be a barrier, because the individual men showed a thoughtfulness towards each other, and focused on their similarities rather than their differences.

Unlike many of the other pieces of work described here, interviews were carried out and recorded with the fathers after the group had finished. Comments from this evaluation include:

There was a good balance between the content being chosen for us and by us.

It was good to have ideas about how to solve things.

The sense of humour was important within the group.

Q. What effect has the group had on you as a father?

Given me insights to what is going on.

Feeling that I am not alone, not the only father in this situation.

Enabling me to see things as I have been too close, not being able to see the wood for the trees.

It helps to have others who do not know you, outside of the family, to talk things through with.

Q. What was it like being in this group?

Little bit nervous the first time.

If you have not been before, you don't know what to expect; the second session was easier and OK.

When the leaders talked about their own experiences, it made it easier for me.

Q. How has your parenting changed?

Little snippets of information that mean that I can think and react, then behave differently towards the children.

I'm not so stuck, I've got another avenue/idea to try.

Makes me look at things from the children's point of view as well as the adult's.

Over the years, Colin has worked with more than 60 fathers within group settings. He says he has learnt a number of important lessons and noticed a number of benefits that have come as a result of this work (both at West Wilts and the previous Family Centre he worked in).

He says: '*Fathers' own evaluations have placed most emphasis on gaining information on child development, on learning the language used by child care agencies and getting ideas and strategies in parenting skills. Fathers have also viewed meeting new people, sharing different points of view, camaraderie and friendship as important factors. Being listened to and communicating with men on a more 'feeling' level and without the fear of competitiveness, put-downs and Mickey-taking ran a close second.*'

Some men described the group as being able to use a different language than at the pub. The majority of fathers said the group had influenced and affected positive change in their parenting skills with their children. Examples of this are, 1 man said he started to enjoy playing with his child, and another said he started reading bedtime stories to his stepchild, which he had not done before.

Outside agencies (in particular Social Services Departments) often report that fathers attend case conferences and meetings more often, and are more assertive and clear about their own and family needs. Local Team managers have reported that early intervention with the fathers had reduced risk and in some cases reduced the need to call a case conference. Health visitors observed fathers who received a service from the Family Centre to be more involved and more confident with their children.

Fathers' comments included:

Q. What was it like being in this group?

You know you're not the only one.

You're not so isolated.

It gets it off your chest.

You find different ways of trying things.

You think of other angles and not just looking through your own windows.

Q. What effect has the group had on you as a father?

It worked: I have stopped smacking my child.

It was difficult for me and my child to look at each other (task at home), but it is working now.

I could tell my child to go upstairs (instead of smacking).

I can think before I act.

Not much change, but I can be more free.

Another group was started on November 2000 with 8 fathers.

As well as these ongoing fathers' groups, Colin has also been running a group for fathers and sons. The aim of this group was to provide boys aged 8-11 years and their fathers, an opportunity to develop a better understanding of the boys' challenging behaviour and for the fathers to implement effective management strategies.

This weekly group met for 8 after-school sessions (4.30pm to 6.00pm), from March to May 2000, with 6 boys and their fathers. It was the sons that were referred, for disruptive behaviour (usually at school, but also often at home), and parents tended to want them 'to be fixed', not really taking responsibility for their behaviour.

Colin's view is that boys' attention-seeking behaviour is often copied from their fathers' behaviour, 'naughty boys have naughty fathers' and that strict authoritarian parenting styles, low confidence, and fathers giving their sons little attention were contributing factors to their disruptive behaviour.

Again, home visits were an important part of the referral process, where an emphasis was placed on including the boys' mother to positively include her in the group; and to gain ideas about what they would like to see changed in the

fathers' and sons' relationship and in particular their sons'.

Sessions had a clear focus, to look at the relationship and interaction between fathers and sons. This was through a series of activities, most of which would last for 15 minutes or so and rarely for longer than 30 minutes. As well as disruptive behaviour, the boys also tended to have poor levels of concentration. They included clay making, trust games, cooking, eye contact games, listening and negotiating exercises, collage making and feelings games. Any exercise that required concentration or reflection were preceded by a 5-minute energetic game, often suggested by the boys themselves.

Two of the fathers said they never played directly with their children and therefore found playing games difficult. Some of the fathers also found it hard to listen to their sons and in accepting that their sons' views might be different from their own. Sometimes fathers dismissed or put down what their sons were saying or became competitive where they thought they always had to be better.

Each boy was given a file, which was used as a diary and was also used for specific homework exercises and overall course aims. Each session started with the participants reporting back about their achievements. Although this activity was specifically for the boys, it became extended to the fathers, especially in relation to controlling their tempers.

A number of lessons were learnt. Colin felt that a pre-meeting with the fathers explaining the purpose of the activities would have reduced some fathers' resistance – as would a more directive approach – and may have helped fathers to focus, especially in the communication activities.

More sessions for fathers to reflect on their own parenting issues may have also supported them to deal with the challenge that the group obviously provided, especially given that most came with the view that the group was for their sons and not themselves.

Again fathers and sons were asked after the sessions, what they thought about it. Comments included:

To fathers:

What effect has the group had on your son?

Short-term none.

Not had any effect on my son at all. He has improved while coming to the group, but he does improve anyway.

He improved his behaviour in the group, he didn't swear or put me down or show off as he usually does. His behaviour also got better at home during the time of the group.

To sons:

What effect has the group had on your dad?

He's changed a lot; my dad has become kinder.

He has grounded me instead of hitting me.

My dad was nicer to me in the group, he listened more and brought me sweets.

To sons:

What effect has the group had on your control of your temper?

Helped me not to lose my temper at school.

I was able to control my temper and not swear at my dad.

To fathers:

What effect has the group had on your control of your temper?

Helped me control my temper more.

Made me look at it in a different way.

Made me want to start smoking again!

Colin says that this is work in progress. They are still trying to find ways that they can offer fathers' and sons' groups, where both can learn and not feel too challenged, in the way that the fathers have to date.

Colin believes a number of lessons have already been learnt from this work, these include:

- The group was most useful where dads were able to attend all sessions with their sons.
- Specific practical activities were most successful. Where activities involved a written or discussion exercise, it was harder to sustain the boys' involvement.
- The age/ability range was too broad to focus on particular or specific issues;
- Many of the parents viewed their children's problems as a result of sibling rivalry; therefore fathers attending the group in some cases involved arranging time off work, leaving their house with their sons and time being spent together (in some cases up to 45 minutes) and this became an important statement to the sons that they were seen as important.

This description was written from a visit and conversation with Colin Holt, one of the fathers' groups and various write-ups, reports and evaluations of the 4 pieces of work described. As these evaluations contained extensive comments from fathers and were carried out by an independent evaluator, most of the fathers' comments were taken from these evaluations.

Colin Holt can be contacted at West Wilts Family Centre, 71 Fore Street, Trowbridge, Wiltshire, and by phone on 01225-751261.

What Works? YMCA 'Dads and Lads'

YMCA Plymouth is a large, well-equipped sports centre, offering fitness-training, sixth form training in sports leadership, outdoor pursuits courses and other community-based programmes. While the Centre is primarily a sports initiative, it also has a strong youth work component. The Centre is the biggest sports facility in Plymouth and has as many as 400, 5-16 year-olds through the door each week, and runs both eleven-a-side teams and five-a-side leagues.

The idea came from Dirk Uitterdijk (YMCA Parenting & Education Support), who suggested that Mark Peard (Programme Director and experienced youth worker), worked with the fathers who tended to bring their sons to the Centre and then left.

Initially there were no specific aims, and the one session a month (on a Saturday evening), was sold as an opportunity for fathers and sons to play football with each other. Saturday night (7pm to 9pm) was thought to be a good time because fathers were less likely to be working, and at home, and once a month meant that the sessions would not disrupt other family activities.

Invitations were sent out in December 1997 to all of those involved in the YMCA football leagues and other Centre activities, the local paper ran an advert and leaflets were distributed as widely as possible. Neither Mark nor David (Centre worker) were confident that they would attract many fathers and sons and were very surprised when 12 dads and 14 lads turned up the first evening.

Teams were quickly selected (mix of dads and lads) and five-a-side games played and, apart from a 15 minute drinks break, games were being played the whole time (which included cricket, frisbee, and hockey). Interestingly, only a couple of the lads were known to the workers, and the sessions appeared to attract those lads who were not so good at football, a couple of whom had bullied their fathers to come to the sessions.

The fathers themselves tended to be mid-30s to mid-40s in age, and while the lads ranged from 8-15, the majority were 12-13 years old. All of the fathers were working and, while there was a mix of professional and manual workers, they all worked noticeably long hours. Not all of the lads were related to the dads; some dads brought their sons and a mate.

While some new fathers and sons came and others went, the numbers continued to attract an average of 12 dads and 14 lads. The drinks breaks provided the workers with an opportunity to talk to fathers about parenting. Both workers were still a bit tentative, but did enough for some of the fathers to talk about specific issues, usually related to their sons' health or behaviour. Relationships were very slow to build up, with football remaining the main focus of the sessions.

The main benefit of these sessions seemed to be the opportunity it gave dads and lads to spend time together doing an activity that they enjoyed. Fathers in jobs where 50-60 hours were the norm, valued the structured sessions that ensured that they spent some time with their sons.

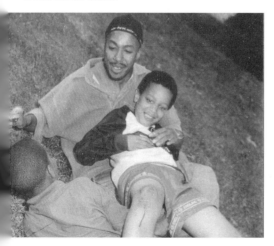

In a review of this initiative, it was reported that 'several (fathers) described the project as totally changing or dramatically improving their relationship with their sons'. This seemed to be because of the structured time and setting that ensured that they were with their boys, at a time when many would expect sons to be wanting more independence from their families. Nothing was known of the relationships fathers had with their sons before this initiative, but their jobs were known to be a massive barrier.

The structured activity also provided lads and dads with an activity to develop their relationships; the boys and young men talked about the sessions as being great fun, enjoyable, and a way to keep fit and one described it as seeing my dad in a normal way, just spending time together and having fun.

It wasn't long before the fathers were requesting that they meet twice rather than once a month. The workers were still hoping to incorporate parenting sessions into the second part of the evening's activities, but this rarely happened. However, an additional evening was arranged, billed as a 'World Cup Night', where apart from the Morocco v Norway game (on the Centre's wide screen TV), and food, a presentation around Rob Parsons' '60-minute father' was offered.

Ten fathers (and one mother) attended this session. The group was split in two and the group leaders commented on how open the parents were to talk about issues relating to the work/life balance. Dave Bruty says that 'the evening showed that parenting issues could be talked about and shared; some fathers borrowed Rob Parsons' video and enjoyed it, asking for more sessions.

This was followed up by additional Saturday morning sessions for fathers to discuss parenting issues. This attracted three or four men on a regular basis, where again Rob Parsons' book were used to provoke discussion. Interestingly, all of the fathers attending these sessions identified specific problems and issues that they were experiencing with their sons.

One was self-harming, another had a genetically based growth problem, another had communication and behaviour issues while the fourth was very concerned about his son's drinking and truanting. Most of the sessions involved reflective discussion, but did seem to fill an important gap for those fathers with concerns about their sons.

These sessions later moved to a Monday night in the pub, but tended to remain rather informal in nature and content. Workers continued to find it difficult to make these sessions more formal or with more participants.

In April 2000, a 'Fun Day' was planned and, while 50 or 60 were expected, over 250 people attended, with more than 120 of these being parents. While the day offered a variety of sport, wall climbing, line dancing and trampoleening and food, it also included a video presentation and discussion about parenting. This was seen as a recruitment opportunity for a planned parenting course.

Twenty eight parents registered for the 6-weekly 2-hour sessions and 12 of these were fathers. Children also came to the sessions and were entertained in the sports hall. All of these men came with their partners and tended to be in full-time work (again working long hours) and often having at least two children. David says that they do not really know why this worked as a recruitment strategy for fathers or whether the more formal (and explicit) approach was a factor.

As a result of the 'Dads and Lads' initiative in Plymouth, and a grant from the Home Office's Family Policy Unit, the YMCA have aimed to replicate and develop this work. Andy Howie (YMCA 'Dads and Lads' project worker) reports that there have been 10 new initiatives; some have taken the football approach, but others such as Fence Houses (in Sunderland) have used angling, Waltham Forest golf, and Reigate have used a variety of sports and activities and also included daughters as well as sons.

Materials have been developed by 'Care for the Family' in Cardiff (based on '60 minute father') and include a glossy 'DAD' magazine with interviews with the likes of Harry Redknapp (manager of West Ham), and more specific fatherhood material.

Andy says that virtually all of the 'Dads and Lads' initiatives have had difficulties in making the transition from a sports and activity focus to a more explicit fathers' programme. Andy believes that this is in part because most of the workers developing these programmes are experienced in sport, although he believes there are some hopeful signs.

In Oswestry (for example), the fathers involved are from a local church and he believes this will help enable the transition. In Chester, a church group of dads are working their way through the 'DAD' material. Cheltenham (who started some2 years ago), held a dads' breakfast and introduced the fatherhood material informally to a small group, and managed a number of discussions which hinged around their relationships with their children, as well as some specific problems such as alcohol use and discipline.

Andy and Dirk have also delivered a workshop for those workers wanting to develop their skills and their confidence in using the materials developed by Care for the Family. They are optimistic that this will help projects to make the transition from activities to delivering explicit fathers' programmes.

In the TSA evaluation of parenting initiatives within the YMCA, a number of components were thought to have been essential to enable the 'Dads and Lads' programmes to be delivered. 'Extensive and well-equipped sports facilities', as was 'enthusiastic and experienced staff who were committed to the project'; 'publicity for the project through the local newspaper' and 'familiarity with the way these programmes have developed'.

Even though the projects have failed to develop the more formal fathers' projects, benefits for both the fathers and sons have been thought to be substantial. They have included:

● providing fathers (often those in work that keeps them away from home for substantial parts of the week) a structured, and enjoyable activity to share with their sons;

● an environment where they can communicate with their sons and other fathers, at a time when fathers and sons are often drifting apart;

● access to parenting help when they are most in need (interestingly those fathers who came forward for the more overt fathers' sessions in Plymouth were those that were very concerned about aspects of their sons' development and behaviour). This would suggest that schemes such as 'Dads and Lads' may prove to be an important point of contact for fathers

for projects that may be of help to them in the future;
- providing an encouraging and caring environment for the young men, and a place they can feel a part of a group;
- improving relationships between the generations and positive male role models.

What the fathers said:

I'm a self-employed landscape gardener, and don't get a lot of time to spend with my boy. The football was something we were both interested in, and both looked forward to it.

We both made new friends, him with other lads that went and I got to know a couple of the dads.

I found the dads'-only meetings helpful, not life changing, but day changing, I think now, before I would have shouted and screamed.

We don't spend much more time together now, but the football gives us both time; we talk.

This description was compiled from conversations with David Bruty (YMCA Plymouth), Andy Howe and Dirk Uitterdijk (YMCA Parenting Project), two fathers and descriptions and evaluation carried out by the Trust for the Study of Adolescence (Innovations in Parenting Support, Debi Roker et. al.) available from the YMCA parenting & education support, Dee Bridge House, 25-27 Lower Bridge Street, Chester CH1 1RS.

What Works? – Emerging themes

The purpose of this publication is to learn from the experience of 10 established fatherhood projects and from the limited literature which has focused on developing practice.

Below, the common themes have been pulled out and offered as important considerations by those wanting to develop new pieces of practice with fathers. Inevitably, within 10 projects, a very broad range of issues emerged, sometimes learning from one contradicted another.

This review has concentrated on issues that appear to be fundamental to developing work with fathers within current practice. Inevitably, some workers offer issues as being fundamental which turn out to be more ideological, or that have a particular 'local' importance; some of these have been discussed, but not included.

At the outset, it was always envisaged that we would concentrate on 'the 10 most important aspects of practice', believing that any more breadth would begin to defeat the object of helping workers reflect on and plan their practice. If we had only presented our view of the 'emerging issues' then I think this would have been inadequate. Instead, we have summarised the 10

examples, to enable workers to see the practice themselves and we have also added contact details, so that the themes that we did not highlight, that are of particular interest to the reader, can be followed up.

Our '10 most important aspects of practice' may, after reading the practice examples, turn out not to be yours, but we have evidenced each of these and think they are crucial to developing practice. However, our experience in supporting work with different groups of men, is that workers reflecting on their practice often leads to an increased confidence and an identification of significant issues, so if that is the outcome, this report has achieved its primary task.

1 Clarity of purpose

Why are we doing what we are doing? What impact do we expect to have on the fathers involved? Work with fathers too often starts with the aim of 'setting up a fathers' group', without so much thought given to what is the purpose of setting up a fathers' group.

A fathers' group without some reflection on what it will do for the fathers involved is very difficult to recruit for. It is no coincidence that by far the majority of fathers' initiatives involve fathers' groups. However, an agency such as Pen Green started with the purpose of reflecting fathers' importance and involving them in the Centre. This led to a fathers' group, but also to a series of initiatives that included staff training, and videoing staff responses to mothers and fathers. Starting with the idea of a fathers' group without thinking through a purpose, narrows thought about appropriate interventions.

The clearer the purpose, the easier it is for fathers to relate and respond. Families Need Fathers stress the importance of offering advice about the court system, to fathers involved in contact and divorce issues; Men United offered support and contact with other fathers looking after their children; the Norwich Young Fathers initially offered a place where young fathers could identify as a group. For some fathers (in the case of 'Man Enough'), they responded to the skills element offered in the courses, at a time when they were having difficulties with their children.

Of course, it is sometimes easier to state a short-term aim, in the case of football for the YMCA Dads and Lads project for recruitment purposes, but the less explicit purpose of offering fathers support and skills development still had to be overcome to engage fathers to the 'fathering' component.

Clarity of purpose has to embody promises made to funders, those issues identified by the organisation, and of course, a purpose that the fathers will respond to. Interestingly, those organisations that would see themselves as 'user-orientated', state their purpose in relation to the client group, while agencies such as Family Centres are more likely to state their purpose in relation to others (child protection), rather than the fathers. 'Work with fathers to make it safer for their partners and children', is a perfectly good purpose, but may lead to difficulties relaying this in a way that fathers will respond to.

2 Reaching fathers

Many fathers do not use services: many men do not use services! Statistically, men do not use GP's surgeries, other primary health care services, dentists (in a preventative way), counselling agencies, libraries, even employment agencies and adult education services as much as women.

Fathers are less involved in children's health, childcare and education services than mothers and less likely to think that agencies expect their involvement. Many professionals have seen this as a reflection of fathers' disinterest in their children, whereas it appears (at least in part), to be fathers' (and men's) reluctance to use a range of services that offer help and support or agencies that are part of a personal preventive strategy.

This has a number of implications for agencies wanting to establish services for fathers. They include that:

- traditional routes used by many agencies (especially other childcare organisations), are less likely to reach fathers. Leaflets to GP's surgeries are less likely to reach fathers than mothers;
- more traditional 'male' routes are worth considering, although very few of the 10 examples did this. Norwich Young Fathers targeted local hostels; FNF used the radio (known to be popular with men) and 'Man Enough' and YMCA, the local media. Other men's initiatives have used sports settings, the Internet and pubs as routes to access men;
- fathers may be best accessed through their partners (if they have one) or their children. Rugby Parents' Centre reached fathers through their partners who were users of the Parents' Centre, and found that they had very little difficulty in recruiting fathers, that is, until they had exhausted this source. They even found that partners sometimes pressured fathers to attend, and staff strongly encouraged mothers to 'lean on' fathers, highlighting to mothers the possible advantages of fathers attending a course (i.e. less tension created by different parenting styles);
- the more contact made with fathers in an informal, but direct way, the

more some fathers responded. 'Man Enough' and FNF were perceived as agencies that were NOT social worker driven, which appeared to help recruitment, while the more 'social work' the agency was, the harder it was to recruit fathers (West Wilts and NEWPIN for example). Sometimes, 'by association' is enough to create a barrier: DIY Dads (a South London fathers' project), funded by the Family Policy Unit of the Home Office, found that some fathers thought, because of its funders that DIY Dads was part of the CSA!, which made fathers reticent to come forward;

- fathers are likely to be reluctant to attend services, whatever agencies offer. Some of the fathers spoken to within the 10 examples, said they were nervous about attending, others said they were terrified, while others had a 'what the hell, let's give it a go' approach. It may be that projects attract men in the latter category, more than the former, so a general approach to life and opportunity, may have a substantial impact on which fathers use services and which ones don't.

Most of the agencies interviewed used a broad net approach to reaching fathers or had a primary source and added to that through other routes. Albert Ford said that 'leaflets about Man Enough' went through the Community

Education magazine, Oxford Parenting Forum, libraries, through partners on other parenting courses, local schools and as fathers came into his Central Oxford shop, he gave them a leaflet and talked to them about the course.'

He estimated that 'a third of the men came via personal contacts (made in his shop), a third from personal contacts through supportive agencies'. FNF, with 25 years' experience, now find that national coverage and word-of-mouth are fathers' main routes to their services. Richard Edmonds (Blackburn and Darwin), recruited via his caseload as a counsellor attached to a GP's surgery, although his target group of fathers was very narrow. As mentioned above, Rugby Parents' Centre recruited via mothers who already used their services, but found that when this source dried up, they couldn't reach enough fathers.

Multi-faceted approaches, via traditional routes for men, and traditional routes for parenting activities; local and national media; word-of-mouth; via partners and agencies own user pool, were all important ways to access fathers. The broader the net, the more likely it is that fathers will be reached.

3 Liking fathers?

All of the examples of practice approached fathers with a positive outlook. They were convinced of the evidence that children benefited from their fathers' involvement; that fathers wanted to be involved and active in their children's lives; that provided with the right environment, fathers were able and willing to reflect on fathering issues and wanted to improve their ability to father their children. Interestingly, while these were the shared beliefs, agencies were not necessarily aware of the evidence to support these assertions.

Even those from agencies that have traditionally had a more negative image, saw fathers 'struggling', 'finding it difficult to cope', and 'needing support' rather than being problematic and disinterested.

Most workers talked about supporting fathers; many of them felt that fathers needed advocates. FNF, Men United and Norwich Young Fathers (MAP, where the group emerged, are also strong advocates for young people), were the most overt about this, while 'Man Enough' and Blackburn and Darwin also saw this as essential, but this occurred on an informal and individual basis.

However, this positive approach and advocacy role often caused some tensions between the fathers' initiatives and others parts of the agencies, or with other organisations. Initiatives were seen as too pro-fathers, assumed sometimes to therefore be anti-mothers and women.

Organisations could be placed on a

spectrum: at one end, there would be FNF and Men United, who are clearly strong advocates for fathers; while at the other end of the spectrum would be West Wilts and Pen Green centres who would state their commitments more around the safety and development of children, rather than being pro-father. The overall purpose of the organisation the fathers' initiative was in could cause tensions.

Interestingly, the tensions for these organisations have emerged in different ways. For FNF (who admit themselves they have some 'radical anti-feminists' within their midst, but strongly believe that they are not prominent within the organisation), there are parenting organisations that are unwilling to work with them, believing that they are anti-women and too much for 'men's rights'.

Men United have also found themselves accused of being anti-women, because they take a pro-father position and inevitably (as is the case for FNF), attract some men with strong views. Men United have sought funding for a Fathers' Centre and male workers, and this has also been seen as anti-women. They have responded by making such comments as: 'But, you women have had a separate project for years, why can't we?, which has confirmed for some that they are anti-women.'

In contrast, centres where children and mothers have been the main users, fathers' initiatives have been seen as

add-ons and often meet at times when the centre is closed, thus avoiding the risks and tensions that may develop.

These issues will need to be managed carefully. Working With Men developed sessions for fathers in a Central London agency that worked with Asian women, who raised concerns about fathers being present, because they had told their husbands that they were going to a centre where there were only women.

These issues are important to manage, but not a reason for avoiding work with fathers. These kinds of tensions inevitably have a bearing on the way that work with fathers develops and will influence the message that agencies and workers project about their view of fathers, to both the fathers themselves and to other agencies.

4 Which fathers?

Most of the 10 examples, defined their service in such a way that would narrow the type of father that came forward. West Wilts, NEWPIN and Blackburn and Darwin were looking for fathers who were struggling to be active, involved fathers. Offering a more therapeutic service, meant that only fathers who were able to acknowledge that they themselves required help and assistance tended to come forward. Initially,

Men United attracted fathers who felt isolated and also tended to be lone fathers with primary care for their children. FNF tended to attract fathers who were in particular circumstances (going through divorce and separation), and 'Man Enough' and Rugby Parents' Centre fathers who were aspiring to being better fathers or who were having difficulties with their anger or disciplining their children. Norwich Young Fathers were, of course, all young (although not teenagers), and YMCA attracted fathers whose sons were keen on football, but not always that good at it.

However, for many of these projects diversity ruled as much as similarity. Children's ages within 'Man Enough' for example, varied from 3-16 years and a similar range could be found in NEWPIN and Rugby Parents' Centre, which often led to smaller groups forming to cater for common interests. Family Centres such as Pen Green and West Wilts, who offered services to specific groups of children, narrowed the target group of fathers.

As work develops further with fathers, specific groups will need to be better understood and targeted. Recent courses developed for expectant fathers (by DIY Dads), has found that this common experience enables short courses to be very closely defined, resulting in a high level of satisfaction for the participants.

5 Recruitment of fathers

Obviously the recruitment of fathers is strongly linked with an agency's ability to contact fathers. However, a number of issues emerged for agencies about the recruitment process, which included:

a) Recruitment took a long time and was labour intensive. Initially, for some of the projects, it took longer to recruit than it took to deliver the course/initiative they planned. There are countless stories of workers becoming enthusiastic about working with fathers, putting out a leaflet, getting no response and concluding that 'there isn't a demand', or 'it is much too difficult'. Because many of the projects relied on word-of-mouth and recommendation from other agencies, this inevitably took time. NEWPIN took 9 months to establish one group. This is unusually long, but agencies have to be prepared for a relatively long lead-in time.

b) Referring agencies were much more hit and miss than most other referral sources. A number of agencies mentioned that shortly after they sent out publicity material, they received calls from the local probation services looking to refer men to a community-based violence programme. Two projects said that local agencies wanted to 'refer the dad from hell' (description of one worker), even though the men were completely inappropriate for the initiative planned.

There were two issues raised here: one was the lack of services targeted at men, leading agencies to consider any service they could refer a man to; and secondly that agencies rarely understood the nature of the provision, or were uneasy and sometimes suspicious because it was for fathers – sometimes assuming that if it was pro-fathers, it must be anti-mothers.

Interestingly some projects, such as West Wilts reported that agencies acting as gatekeepers for the fathers they were in contact with, needing to be convinced of the value of the provision, before they would consider referral. So, the two extremes often co-existed, fathers' projects being used as a dumping ground for fathers others couldn't, or didn't want to work with, or agencies needing to be convinced that 'their' fathers would be alright.

West Wilts worked hard at informing potential referring agencies about what fathers would and wouldn't get, and organised lunches and short seminars, which also raised awareness of fathering issues.

c) A number of projects used the local media (especially the radio and press) to reach fathers directly. Interestingly, all of these said that the media were sympathetic to their initiatives. Articles in the Oxford local press concentrated on Albert Ford's 'colourful past', but positively conveyed the values of the project, while the Plymouth Press concentrated on the activity base of the YMCA project.

The Norwich local press included coverage of both the handbook the group produced, and of the young fathers' lives. Some agencies have shied away from the local media because of their experience of poor reportage of such issues as child protection or sexual abuse. However, the 10 projects' experience of the local media was that they were enthusiastic, sympathetic and very valuable as a route to contacting fathers directly.

d) Most of the agencies provided specific, relatively short-term programmes, so recruitment was an ongoing issue. Those that provided longer-term initiatives also said that recruitment remained a problem. Fathers moved on, their circumstances changed, they got jobs or went on courses, or they decided that their involvement in the fathers' projects had run its course. Men United and Norwich Young Fathers both said that they had difficulties recruiting new fathers to the initiative. The closeness and levels of support offered by fathers to each other sometimes created a barrier for new fathers coming in, or levels of expectation became too high for new fathers to feel comfortable.

6 What are you offering?

Interestingly, content, style and approach showed the broadest range within the 10 examples: NEWPIN providing a therapeutically-based 35 week programme, through to (sometimes) one-off attendance at a self-help group with FNF; 'Man Enough' structured, skills-based programme; Blackburn and Darwin's social skills format; Pen Green ongoing fathers' groups with a range of other initiatives aiming to get fathers more involved in the Centre's day-to-day activities; YMCA and a sports-base leading to discussion-based initiatives; MAP with its strong advocacy stance; and Men United using a community development model of working, mixed with an advocacy model.

Reflective exercises, role-play, tasks to complete, were all common, and many of the projects did not necessarily confine their discussions to fathering issues, Men United looked at men's health, Pen Green violence, feminism and men's friendships, obviously related, and always having implications for fathers, but what doesn't?

What appeared to be more important than content, methods, styles and form was that they related to the purpose. Those projects where purpose was less specific, the more fathers questioned methods, style and form. So, for example Pen Green's ongoing fathers' group often discussed style and form, but rarely purpose and sometimes there were sub-groups of fathers who were looking for (and sometimes getting) different benefits. This causes problems for those organisations that see the work as 'more organic', and developmental.

Both Men United and MAP went through different phases, where the focus (and indeed the purpose) changed. In both cases they started as support groups, and in the case of Men United they became more of a research, advocacy and campaigning group. Norwich Young Fathers followed a similar path, producing their handbook, which again some enjoyed and others found less relevant to their needs.

7 Why would they want to get involved?

Understanding the motivation for fathers' involvement was central to many of these projects' success in both recruiting and meeting the needs of fathers. Timing was often critical, as fathers rarely talked about having known of the project for ages and just not getting around to it. Much more often it was a quick decision, a timely conversation or a crisis and sometimes what James Levine refers to as 'golden opportunities'.

There were 3 levels of motivation recurrently mentioned: societal changes, others' expectations and fathers' own needs.

Societal changes have led to dramatic developments in the labour market where fathers have traditionally been the ones more likely in full-time employment, earning enough to keep themselves and their families. Employment patterns have led to a very diverse set of arrangements within families, from fathers still the primary bread-winners through to mothers being the only bread-winners.

This has had a knockdown effect on families and childcare roles and responsibilities, leading to some men working even more hours (often out of anxiety of losing their jobs or poor pay levels), while others have grown into the role of primary carers for their children. Some families have made these changes through choice, while others, because of the employment options, have been forced to review roles and responsibilities.

Others' expectations have often been as a result of employment changes. Men's partners (certainly if they have taken the bread-winner role), reasonably expect fathers to take the role that is left. Fathers often came forward saying that they felt guilty because they did not spend enough time with their children, or that their partner thought that the course would be a good idea, or that 'society expects us to do it now'.

Sometimes others' concerns, particularly about sons' underachievement and possible waywardness (drugs, criminal activity etc.), had led fathers to explore their relationships with their sons and grapple with their 'role modelling'.

Fathers' own needs, are often motivated by either of the two above, or what

fathers often express as 'I want to be a better father than my own'. Generations of bread-winning have often left fathers talking about their own fathers as distant, not emotionally available, absent and too much of a disciplinarian.

Fathers will say that they do not want to make the 'mistakes' that their fathers did. They don't want to be 'the tiger in the house', and want to be 'able to talk to their children'. That being out of the workplace has left them isolated, that they never learnt to be a father, and that they were concerned that they would lose their relationship with their children (because of divorce and separation), are also often mentioned.

Projects all succeeded in relating to these motivations and constructed programmes and initiatives to respond to them. The YMCA found that most of the fathers involved in their 'Dads and Lads' programmes were working full-time (and often more) and were increasingly concerned that they were not spending time with their sons.

The structured fun activities fitted the bill perfectly for them. Rugby Parents' Centre fathers were usually motivated by their concerns about the quality of their relationships with their children (often reinforced by their partners). 'Man Enough' also attracted fathers who were motivated by their own impatience and anger towards their children.

FNF fathers were motivated by their critical situations, but this was compounded by other (the Courts' and solicitors') views that they were not competent to look after or be significant in their children's lives. Recognition of the importance of the fathers' role and the expectations of staff that fathers would get involved, led to Pen Green's success in involving fathers.

The more we understand these motivations and which fathers are motivated by what, the more likely we are to recruit and work effectively with individual fathers.

8 Workers' skills, and attitudes

Diversity reigns within the workers that delivered the 10 projects: family workers, social workers, community workers, trainers, advice workers, students and volunteers. Almost all of the staff involved in delivery were male and almost all were fathers. It would be easy to conclude that this was work that only fathers could do, and if not fathers than at least men, but this would be a little hasty.

We may be able to conclude that fathers are more likely to have the knowledge, motivation, commitment, skills and attitudes that workers need, but only by exploring the type of skills and attitudes required to develop this work. The comments below have been drawn from both the views of workers interviewed and those fathers who made comments about the initiatives.

Knowledge of fathering, fathers, their motivation and experience appear to be the main components that workers need. Knowledge is, of course, not gender specific; however, in some circumstances, such as in FNF, experience of being male within the family court system does seem to be central to the service delivered.

Motivation and commitment to develop and sustain work with fathers appeared to be essential. Some of the workers interviewed had themselves been involved for a number of years, sometimes with very low budgets, sometimes having to deal with reluctance from their own or other agencies and with a range of challenges, not least from the fathers themselves.

Again, motivation is not gender specific; however, wider perceptions of fathers as a group, personal experience of fathering and the barriers that may be placed between them and their active involvement, are likely to be stronger for men who are fathers. Sometimes motivation and commitment are barriers for some women (and indeed men). Poor experiences of fathers (their own and their children's), and wanting to sort out fathers, because of the negative attitude they are seen as having on children, can create barriers for work to develop.

Skills and attitudes varied enormously within the 10 examples of practice, but some stand out. A positive attitude towards fathers was by far the strongest, a comfort in talking/asking about fathering and about fathers' experience was also significant. A number of fathers mentioned workers being understanding and 'knowing' what they were going through. 'Knowing' did not necessarily refer to knowledge, but a combination of being sympathetic, having heard it before, and issues not needing to be described in a lot of detail.

Fathers made comments such as 'he knew the tensions between work and bringing up your family'. Obviously there is a fine line between 'knowing' and making assumptions, but fathers described this quality a lot. Is this gender-specific? Even if it isn't for the worker, it may be for the fathers themselves. Gender assumptions about what can be understood pervade, with books such as Women are from Venus and Men are from Mars trying to explain/or play on assumptions that we don't and sometimes can't 'understand' each other.

Some fathers, initially, especially if they are hesitant to attend the project, may jump to a series of assumptions based on the person's gender and experience. Young women (who are not mothers), are likely to be seen as the least able to 'understand' and 'know' even if they do!

A number of fathers validated the ability of workers to enable them and others to talk, and often mentioned how much they learnt from other fathers, rather than the workers themselves. This may mean that creating environments where fathers can talk and reflect may be much more important than being an expert. In fact, a number of fathers said that they appreciated workers who did not 'know it all', and that they were 'not experts'. Workers being experts often led fathers to think they would be judged, which usually meant judging as not good enough. Again this is not gender specific.

Fathers' preferences are not really known. We failed to asked fathers whether they thought mothers/women could have worked on the programmes/initiatives, but when men are asked about their preferences for the gender of the professional, it is not as clear-cut as when women are asked.

So, for example, eight out of ten women state a preference for a female doctor if given a choice. In contrast, four out of ten men say they would prefer a male doctor, the same for a female doctor and two out of ten say they don't mind as long as they are competent.

This suggests that the gender of the worker may not be as significant for men as it appears to be for women. Homophobia (the fear of other men), as well as socialisation encouraging men to seek comfort and emotional outlets with women, may in fact make some women (with the appropriate knowledge, motivation, commitment, skills and attitudes), more able to develop this work.

It is too early (in the development of fathers' work), to jump to hasty conclusions about fathers being the only (or indeed the best) people to develop this work, but an exploration of who fits the bill and what fathers may respond to could be timely.

9 Fathers are men too

A number of the 10 projects went much further than discussing with men their role as fathers, indeed in many cases the fathers requested it. The most obvious are Men United and their men's health course and Pen Green's men's group, who looked at a range of topics that had implications for being a father, but would have been more recognisable in a men's group. The same process seems to occur in mothers' groups where 'mother' and 'women' would be addressed simultaneously and sometimes seamlessly.

The YMCA worked on the basis that fathers with sons would be attracted to a football initiative, while NEWPIN had to take into account that their more therapeutic approach required men to be prepared to do more non-traditional male activities (such as talk about themselves, reflect on and discuss their emotional lives). Inevitably, they attracted those men who had had this experience before and found it useful. Examples such as Men United and MAP had to move the fathers involved into a more reflective style, so an

understanding of men and any reluctance there may be to go below their 'masculine fronts', was essential for workers to both understand and grapple with, if the work was to develop.

Stereotypes and strong assumptions about men were as important to understand and question, as those about fathers. Many people still believe that men are unable or unwilling to express their emotions, are unable or unwilling to explore their roles as men and as fathers. If these assumptions were held by the 10 examples, this work would not have developed. They would have never managed (or in fact wanted) to get men into the room in the first place.

10 Increasing fathers' use of mainstream services

This last theme did not emerge from the 10 examples, but as a result of writing about them. Contacting, recruiting and engaging fathers is likely to continue to be an important issue in years to come. These difficulties are compounded by some men's reluctance to use support and prevention services. A number of the 10 examples of practice found difficulties in sustaining both the initiatives, but also fathers' involvement.

Men United, for example, found recruiting new fathers difficult, and believed that creating a 'Fathers' Centre', a 'centre of our own' was the way to overcome this difficulty. The rationale for this is often that professionals and agencies are not 'male or father-friendly', which is certainly the case in too many agencies.

As we have discussed above, too often inexperienced workers think about a men's group before they think about purpose. This frame of mind that says that fathers want and need separate provision, may send us off in one direction, whereas developments may have to happen in this and the opposite. Working With Men have recently been funded for a worker who will spend half of their time developing initiatives that respond to local fathers' needs (in a South London SureStart initiative) and half of their time supporting other SureStart initiatives to integrate fathers. This is based on a view that separate initiatives is a very important short-term aim, while in the longer term, mainstream agencies' views of fathers and fathers' views of mainstream services have to change.

A valuable component of fathers' initiatives is the need to challenge men's attitudes towards support services and help-seeking, and also mainstream agencies' attitudes towards fathers and men generally. If we are effective in this, separate provision for fathers will be a necessity of the past, and 'male unfriendly' services the same.

Summary of findings

Over the last 25 years, there have been scattered pieces of practice that have rarely been recorded, let alone evaluated. This report started from the assumption that those wanting to develop new pieces of work can learn from existing practice.

From the analysis of existing, established projects, there were 10 common themes identified as significant reasons why these projects worked. They were:

- Projects were very clear (or became clear) about their purpose.

- Fathers were reached when a multi-faceted targeting approach was used.

- Agencies were 'father positive' and communicated that to both fathers and other agencies.

- Agencies knew which fathers they were targeting and knew something about them.

- Projects recognised that recruitment of fathers took time and needed to be sustained.

- Agencies knew what they were offering and communicated that to fathers.

- Projects understood what motivated fathers to get involved.

- There were identifiable skills, and attitudes common in project workers.

- Agencies realised that fathers were men too, and adapted programmes and recruitment strategies to take this into account.

- While projects did not identify it, we concluded that agencies needed to increase fathers' use of mainstream services.

Trefor Lloyd
Working With Men
June 2001

Appendix 1

Established fathers' projects initially contacted

1   Young Fathers' Group, MAP, Norwich

2   Blackburn Fathers' Group

3   NEWPIN, South London

4   Man Enough, Oxford

5   Men United, Nottingham

6   HMYOI Deerbolt, County Durham

7   Rugby Parents' Centre, Rugby

8   Parent Network, Glasgow

9   Fathers Plus, Newcastle Upon Tyne

10   Families Need Fathers, London

11   Pen Green Family Centre, Corby

12   Lawrence Weston Family Centre, Bristol

13   West Wilts' Family Centre, Trowbridge

14   YMCA, Plymouth

15   A Dad's Place, Newcastle-Upon-Tyne

16   Sheffield Children's Centre, Sheffield

17   Stonewall Gay Dad's Group, London

18   'Canny Lads', Longbenton, Newcastle Upon Tyne

19   Biker Sands Family Centre, Newcastle-Upon-Tyne, NE6 2FF

20   Tiddlers & Toddlers, London

21   Teams Family Centre, Newcastle-Upon-Tyne

22   Aylesbury YOI, Berkshire

23   Ormistan Trust, Suffolk

Appendix 2

What works? Interview schedule

Where did the idea come from?

Were fathers asking for the service?

Who wanted it and why?

Who was involved?

Was it funded from the beginning?

Who did the work?

What were the aims then?

How did you get fathers involved?

What did you learn through this process?

How did others react to this work? (enthusiastic/resistant)

How has it developed since then?

How has it changed?

What has happened about funding? (more secure, less secure)

What do you think fathers have gained? (individually and collectively)

Has that changed since you started?

What is the future of the project?

Who is involved now?

What skills have the workers developed?

What would you say to a project just starting out?

What were the three main challenges for your project?

What have been the three most important things you have done right?

What are the three most pronounced mistakes you have made?

Has the project been evaluated?

Thank you for your time.